T0407838

Dr Clara Doran

HEADS UP

HOW TO LOOK AFTER YOUR BRAIN SO IT WILL LOOK AFTER YOU

For both my Michaels.

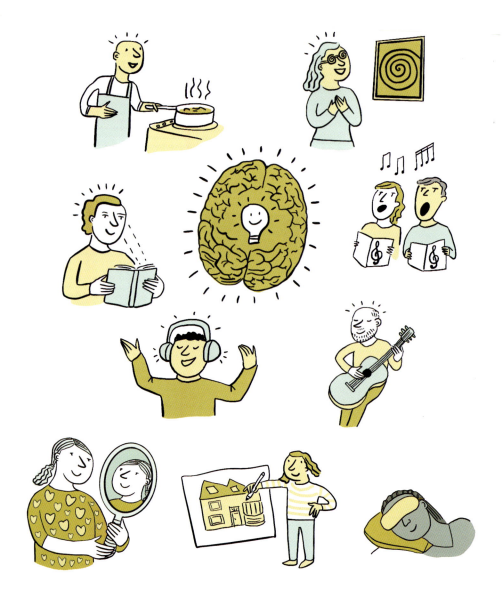

Dr Clara Doran

HEADS UP

HOW TO LOOK AFTER YOUR BRAIN SO IT WILL LOOK AFTER YOU

Leaping Hare Press

CONTENTS

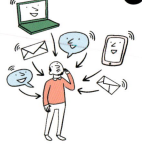

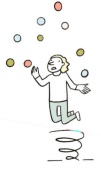

Introduction
6

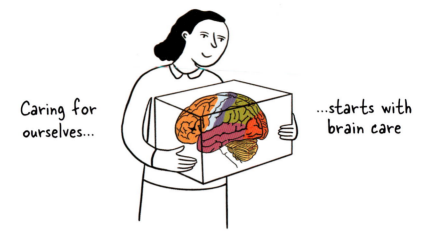

Caring for ourselves...

...starts with brain care

Dear Reader,

This is a book about you.

Funny, amazing, exhausted you.

By picking this up you have already chosen to do something to care for yourself, and for that I want to say well done (and thank you).

When we care for ourselves, everything else in our lives works better.

But here's the secret that not enough people know.

Caring for ourselves starts with brain care.

By the time we have worked through these thirteen lessons together, you will see why.

Don't let the word 'brain' put you off. Yes, they might be gross to look at, but our brains are amazing, undervalued and most importantly, they make us who we are. The good, the bad and the ugly bits of ourselves are all connected to our brain and how it functions.

And here is the best bit – we can change both the way our brain functions and all the many outputs that come as the result of that.

We can do this at any stage of our lives. (I had a patient who went to university at eighty to take a second degree!)

As well as finding ways to make the everyday better, there will be times in life when we really need a way out, or through, what we cannot even begin to see.

These lessons are to help you feel informed and ready to get through those tricky times as best as you can.

How do I know this?

I have been seeing patients for more than twenty years and nearly everything I have learnt about health and life has come from the privilege of caring for them. Somewhere in the middle of that, I became a patient with a lifelong incurable brain condition myself. In parallel, I became a mother to a little boy with blond hair that looked like he was permanently plugged into a socket and a laugh that could extinguish every worry I'd ever had.

As I navigated my new life as a mother, patient and doctor, how I'd lived before my diagnosis didn't work anymore. It took me a few years and further study of health (and myself) to understand why, and that I could improve how I felt.

In my doctor life, when I was putting together patients' symptoms with blood results and the stories they would tell me about their lives, I always viewed health as a jigsaw puzzle, one that can take a full lifetime to get all the pieces in place.

What I've realised from being a patient, and the current research into brain health, is that our brain, and all its brilliance, forms the corners and edges of that puzzle.

We have to start with these pieces to begin to help everything else make sense.

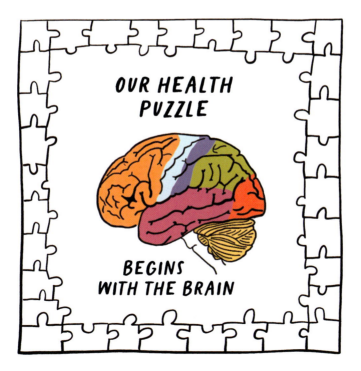

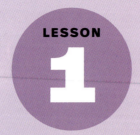

LESSON

1

STOP, LOOK, LISTEN

Before we get started, I'm going to ask you a question. There is no right or wrong answer, (don't panic), and if you don't have any answers that is OK, too. I'm going to help you figure it out.

HOW DO YOU FEEL IN YOURSELF?

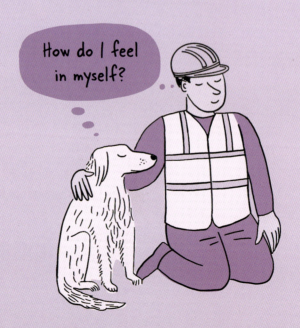

If you have an answer, keep it in your head or write it down. You can say more than one thing.

Before we look under the hood of that answer, I want to come clean. I've asked that question to patients thousands of times in my career as a GP. If I had kept a tally of the replies I received, I know that there would have been four main answers.

'Tired'   'I don't know'   'Fine'
'That's what I'm here to find out'

Given that the number of physical symptoms listed on a symptom tracker is 28, and the number of emotions we can experience is calculated to be somewhere between 12 and 34,000, I have always been aware that these answers seemed vague and non-specific.

When I became a patient myself, I tried multiple times to ask myself that question. And I realised *it's a really hard question to answer.*

IF YOU DON'T REALLY KNOW HOW YOU FEEL, HOW CAN YOU MAKE ANYTHING BETTER?

I have a tried-and-tested method for getting in touch with how I feel. I call it STOP, LOOK, LISTEN

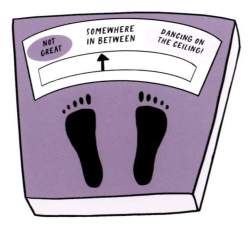

CHECK IN WITH HOW YOU FEEL DAILY

STOP

This is the hardest bit.

Between everything that is going on, both within and around us, it is easy to lose ourselves somewhere in the middle.

If the car you were driving was spinning out of control, you wouldn't think of looking under the hood when the engine and wheels were still running.

So, stop.

LOOK

Paying attention to our daily habits and routines and how they make us feel can be incredibly helpful.

Understanding what and why we do things can help us decide how they are impacting us, positively or negatively.

So, look.

LISTEN

You've heard this one before. Whether you call it a gut feeling, Spidey sense or your intuition, it's there to help us make the choices and decisions that are right for us.

My favourite examples are:

'IT'S HARD TO DESCRIBE, DOCTOR, BUT I JUST KNOW SOMETHING ISN'T RIGHT.'

This can be the opening line of the simplest or most complex of consultations. In my experience it has more than once even led to a cancer diagnosis.

'WHEN YOU FIND THE RIGHT ONE, YOU WILL JUST KNOW.'

We say this to each other when we are looking for a place to live, a partner to love or even the perfect winter coat. And it's frustratingly true.

So, listen to yourself.

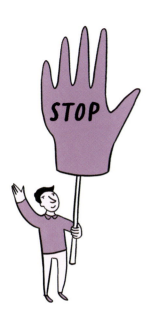

STOP

STEP 1: Eliminate distraction and let whatever thoughts appear be there.

What comes to your mind? Shopping list? To dos? Everything you forgot to do yesterday? Me, too. But, once you weed out all the practical stuff, what are you left with?

STEP 2: Body Scan

Picture yourself in an airport security scanner and work your way up from your toes to your hair. Hopefully you can glide through this quickly and feel that you have no areas of concern. But if you do, pause and take a mental note where something doesn't feel quite right.

STEP 3: Mind Scan

Is your energy high or low? Do you feel comfortable and content with this feeling? Or not? Can you drift into a relaxed but alert state, aka 'quiet wakefulness'?

Research shows that this state can help us work through complex thoughts and possibly reinforce recent learnings. This process can help with our brain cells' ability to reshape themselves based on learnings and experiences, a process known as 'plasticity'.

If your mind goes blank when you think like this, it could mean one of two things. Having a clear mind – a conscious state of thoughtlessness – is the meditation holy grail. If this is what happens to you when you pause to check in with yourself and how you feel, congratulations . . . keep going!

Alternatively, though, you may be frozen. When your mind is a complete blur and you can't think of anything, this might be symptom of feeling anxious or being overwhelmed. Don't try to think of answers. Focus on breathing exercises and taking time to pause for yourself.

Sitting quietly, breathing and trying to focus on yourself might send you into a tailspin. If that's you right now, ask yourself more practical things – what am I enjoying at the moment? What am I worrying about? Looking forward to? When was the last time I felt really happy or positive? What was I doing and who was around me at the time? (Maybe you were on your own and that was what brought you pure bliss.)

Starting to ask yourself these questions can be hard, and feels a bit weird, at first.

Think about how you would sound if you asked your child or someone you cared about these questions. Alternatively, hearing them come from a trusted voice might make it easier to listen to and answer. Choose your favourite caring TV Doctor voice or a narrator from a podcast or audiobook you love and see how that feels. For me, it's Meryl Streep (as herself, not Miranda Priestly . . .)

STEP 4: Practise
Taking even a minute or two to think about how we feel may feel weird. But the more we practise becoming aware of ourselves like this, the better and easier it will feel.

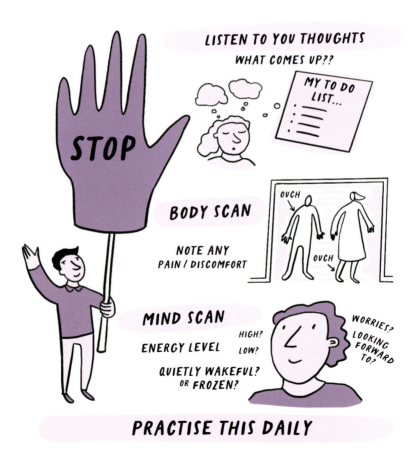

Box breathing

Conscious breathing can help you get to grips with any situation. The box breathing technique is the quickest, and easy to do in public without anyone noticing.

- Breathe in for a count of four
- Hold for a count of four
- Exhale for four
- Pause for four
- Repeat

When we do this even a handful of times, we *slow down our heart rate* and nervous system, which gives us time to actually pay attention.

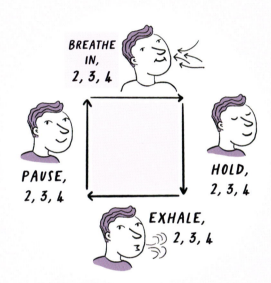

LOOK

When we take a moment to look around us, there are distractions and confusing messages everywhere. This can make it extremely challenging to notice what is really happening within us, and how our environment is impacting this.

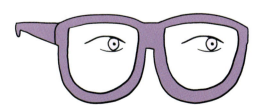

Take a moment to look through your browsing history. Then, if you use social media take a few more minutes to review the last few things you watched. Finally, move to email and your text or WhatsApp messaging threads.

I can guarantee that if you were to write down the last five threads from each of these different sources, you'll find you are jumping between topics as if the floor was lava.

This is life now. And it may be necessary to have the multiple different threads you are weaving together to make your everyday tick. But it's not without consequences.

Your brain was not built to juggle immediate responses required from your boss, three different WhatsApp groups, finding a reliable plumber, laughing at politicians, being shown social media ads *and* dealing with your mother ALL AT THE SAME TIME.

THE GOAL IS LEARNING TO GROUND YOURSELF IN WHAT IS REAL FOR YOU

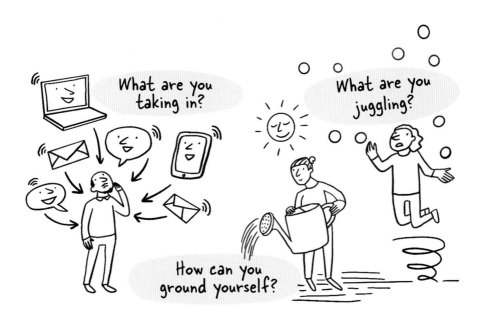

Negativity Bias

Our brains' sole function is to keep us alive. Detecting threats is an essential way this survival mechanism works, so the more bad stuff we are aware of, the more our brain hunts out on its mission to keep us away from possible danger.

Want to stay aware but not constantly panicked? Limit \ how often you watch the news or read less than positive news stories. Notice how you feel and react after reading them and adjust how and when you read these articles accordingly.

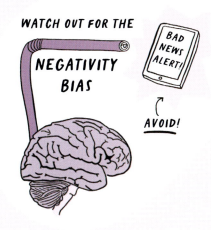

WATCH OUT FOR THE

NEGATIVITY BIAS

BAD NEWS ALERT!

AVOID!

With so much to be frustrated and sad about, it's easy to react to everything. This reaction may occur internally even when we don't say it to anyone. While we might think we then just move on with our day, the responses in our cells say differently. Consuming bad news can trigger emotional and physical stress responses, both of which can negatively impact our health.

ARE THERE ANY RED FLAGS?

LISTEN

Thankfully our bodies and minds are the perfect place to start trying to work out what is happening within. They can tell us how we are in ourselves when we are able to listen.

Physical warning signs:

Changes in appetite

Physical ability and energy

Persistent or recurrent aches and pains

Sleep disturbances

Skin breakouts or dryness

Heart racing

Feeling sweaty

Toilet habits – pay attention to frequency, discomfort and changes to wees or poos

Weight changes – up, down or a bit of both

Hair thinning

Periods – variations in regularity, flow, pain, cyclical symptoms

Mental Health warning signs:

Irritability

Exhaustion

Apathy

Lack of enjoyment

Decreased tolerance of little things that go wrong – road rage is an excellent barometer for stress

Acting out of character, for example, getting in a flap about things that never used to bother you

Running late when you used to be a stickler for time

Everything Changes

Now that we've got some ideas on where we are starting from, something to remember is that things change all the time. We have approximately 60,000 thoughts a day, so how you feel in yourself will change too.

Proactively getting into the habit of asking yourself 'Hang on, how am I doing/ feeling today?' at least daily, is a good idea. Don't wait for the day to go belly up to check in because the way you feel when everything is going wrong is probably stressed/ bad/annoyed. Remember that negativity bias? When there is troublesome stuff going on, it's hard to see anything beyond that as our brain is in survival mode.

What matters about this is that **tuning into yourself needs to become a regular habit**.

ONLY WHEN WE KNOW HOW WE FEEL WITHIN OURSELVES, DO WE KNOW WHEN SOMETHING IS REALLY OFF AND NEEDS ACTION.

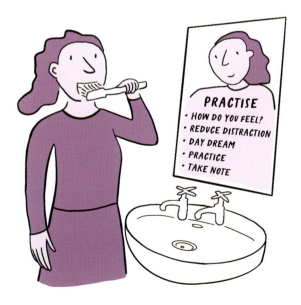

SLEEP, NAP, REST

Sleep remains one of the biggest mysteries
of our human lives. Why do we do it? Do
you need it? And why is getting a good
night's sleep so incredibly difficult?

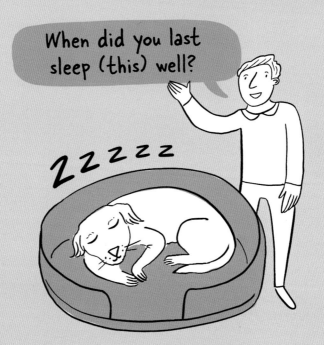

When did you last
sleep (this) well?

ZZZZZ

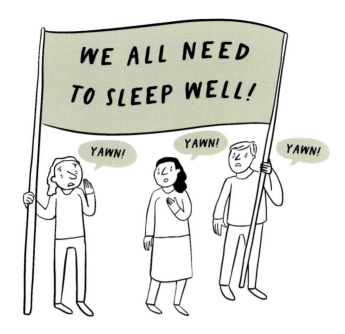

Steven, a patient I saw on and off for about six years, was obsessed with sleep. 'I've never slept well,' he told me, 'even as a kid I was uninvited to sleepovers because I was always awake too much and the other kids (and their parents) hated it.'

He was adamant he couldn't sleep more than two hours in a row, then he'd wake and either take something or do something and then sleep for another two hours. Sometimes he just got up around 4.30 a.m. and got on with his day.

I'd ask him if he needed to nap in the daytime or go to bed early, but he always said no. No matter what time he got up or went to bed, it was always the same. He was seeing me because he was exhausted (unsurprisingly) and he wanted to know why he couldn't sleep properly.

Spoiler: I didn't know the answer but I knew I needed to understand more to help Steven. And I knew he wasn't alone in his nocturnal adventures.

Why do we sleep?

Sleeping is a key biological process, like breathing or blinking, and it is something that we require to stay alive. You could die of sleep deprivation before you die of

We have an in-built drive to sleep that cannot be switched off. However, the quality of our sleep is also influenced by our natural (circadian) rhythms. You will know this if you've ever taken a long-haul flight and wake up hungry at 3 a.m. or can't stay awake past sunset.

Think of sleep as your brain (+hormones + your immune system) working the nightshift in a busy airport. If that essential night-time work doesn't get done, things might not run quite so smoothly and on time the next day. In the wee small hours, your brain cells become a deep-cleaning, re-stocking, hormone-managing night staff.

Hormones From the release of brain-communicating chemical messengers to essential growth hormones in the earliest years of life, your brain at night is the room where this happens.

Deep clean Metabolic waste products are broken down from cells and cleaned out overnight to keep brain cells (neurons) healthy. The protein amyloid is one of these waste products that is efficiently broken down at night. High levels of amyloid in the brain are associated with increased risk of Alzheimer's disease.

Immune function One reason you keep getting sick might be because you aren't sleeping enough to help your immune system do its job. Research has shown that people who were given a dose of a live cold virus were four times more likely to develop symptoms if they regularly had fewer than six hours of sleep per night versus those who had more than seven hours of zzzz.

Cognitive function Disrupted sleep can reduce your brain cells' ability to rest and regenerate. This can impact language processing so your speech can become slurred or it can be harder to find the words you are looking for when you're sleep-deprived.

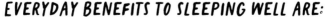

EVERYDAY BENEFITS TO SLEEPING WELL ARE:

Better mood and improved resilience

Better relationships

More successful

Better health

What's the time? Your brain knows

Our genes provide operating instructions for every cell in our body to do their job. How our cells process this information, and how efficiently they do their job is impacted by our bodies' natural rhythms. This circadian rhythm is controlled primarily by the master clock in your brain – a specialised group of around 20,000 cells known as the SCN. Key to its function is communication with other organs responsible for hormone production, including growth hormone. Think of it as your sleep centre remote control.

What helps your SCN drive falling sleep, waking up and flick between hormone production channels and organ communication? Light.

When specialised cells within the SCN detect light or dark (or blue light – more on that later) this triggers those important hormones and clock settings in other organs to switch on or off.

By understanding the key biological efffect of light on our natural rhythms, we can impact how and when we sleep, and subsequently our digestion, stress responses and mood.

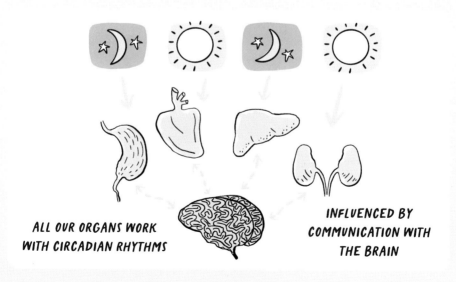

ALL OUR ORGANS WORK WITH CIRCADIAN RHYTHMS

INFLUENCED BY COMMUNICATION WITH THE BRAIN

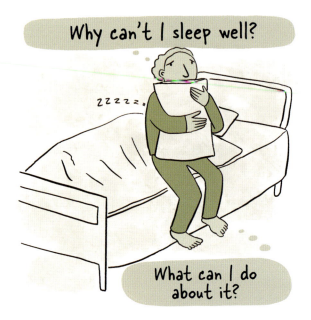

Why are so many of us struggling to sleep well?

Sleep is essential for life, requires minimal effort or equipment and is usually quite enjoyable – so what's going wrong?

Poor mental health It's impossible to have good mental health if you don't sleep well. But the issue with that is that a symptom of mental health disorders is disordered sleep. Here we have the perfect example of the chicken vs the egg.

We've never learnt to 'sleep well' We just go to bed and expect that we can sleep. Imagine going to your fridge and thinking your dinner would just land on your plate. Nope – you have to think about it, shop for it, prepare and cook it THEN eat it. Sleep needs TLC too.

MLS – Modern Life Sabotage Whether you are a serial Netflixer, marathon training at midnight or just sending that one last email to your boss, these 'essentials' of modern life are a death knell to a good night's sleep.

We are worrying about sleeping Have you ever slept well the night before you have an early flight, an exam or a big presentation? When we need and want it the most, sleep can be at its most elusive. One reason for that is the worry factor. By knowing this and looking at our sleep behaviours with a close-up lens, we can make changes.

What can we do to improve our sleep?

Before we get into sleep prep, remember these three things.

First, nights of bad sleep will be part of our lives. That's OK and totally normal.

What we need is to have the tools in place to help us ride that storm of sleeplessness and know we can break out of it back into better sleep when we are ready.

Second, your body and mind tell you when you are tired – pay attention!

Third, when you are in a phase of feeling tired, daytime tools can be helpful sticking plasters to restoring a sense of balance, calm and energy.

THE BASICS

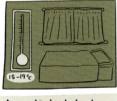

A cool, dark bedroom

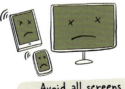

Avoid all screens 1–2hrs before bed

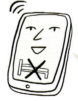

Keep me away from your bed!

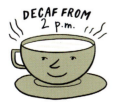

DECAF FROM 2 p.m.

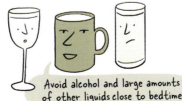

Avoid alcohol and large amounts of other liquids close to bedtime

Sleep school: troubleshooting

Work backwards What time is it realistic for you to go to bed? That may seem an obvious question, but so many of us have unrealistic expectations. The question isn't when you are going to bed, it is what you need to do *before* you can go to bed. I have fallen into this trap so many times it's embarrassing. 'I'm going to bed tonight at 9 p.m.', I say to my husband as we sit down to dinner at 7.30. If you set a bed time then miss it, this can trigger a negative thought cycle and more self-sabotaging behaviours. Let's aim for 10.30 instead and work from there.

Wind down If we prepare for sleep like we prepare for going to work, we are giving ourselves the best chance possible to sleep well. Actively winding down might be reading, journaling, stretching or meditation – all proven to help improve sleep quality and help you fall asleep faster. Baths – yes or no? If you choose yes, *not* too hot *or* too close to bed – they can have the opposite effect.

Routine Our bodies crave routine, so ideally we should be planning for bedtime and wake up time as the same most days. However, listening to how you feel matters too. The optimal goal is to be tired when you go to bed so you fall asleep easily.

Don't lie awake in bed Your bed should be a place of calm, quiet and respite from the stresses of the day. If you put your head on the pillow and start to have an outpouring of worries running through your head, these thoughts can set off your sympathetic nervous system and trigger a fight-or-flight reaction, meaning adrenaline starts pumping and you become more awake than ever.

When this happens, it's time for an intervention.

If you go to bed and can't sleep after twenty minutes, then the answer is to get up. Consider it a false start.

Go and do something else for thirty minutes and enjoy what you are doing. Then go back to bed and try again. Keep repeating this cycle until you fall asleep. And do it tomorrow night too. Eventually, you will retrain yourself that bed is for sleep and when your head hits the pillow, you will fall asleep faster.

Notebook by the bed

It's 2 a.m. and you remember you didn't do THAT THING yesterday. You are kicking yourself and thinking how and when you can fit that into tomorrow. One thing is sure, lying awake worrying about it isn't going to help you: a) do it, or b) get back to sleep.

When that happens, and it will, a notebook or pad of sticky notes by the bed is the perfect thing to help you scribble it down, get it off your mind, and fall back to sleep.

Sleep mask

Ever tried to sleep in broad daylight on a plane? Darkness tells our brain that it's time to sleep. You can help that by wearing a sleep mask.

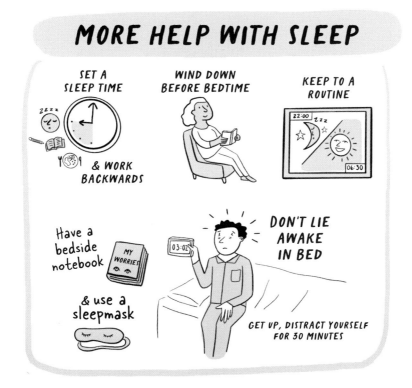

MORE HELP WITH SLEEP

SET A SLEEP TIME
zzzz
& WORK BACKWARDS

WIND DOWN BEFORE BEDTIME

KEEP TO A ROUTINE
22:00 zzz
06:30

Have a bedside notebook
MY WORRIES
03:02
DON'T LIE AWAKE IN BED

& use a sleepmask

GET UP, DISTRACT YOURSELF FOR 30 MINUTES

Sleep School: day-time helpers

You slept badly but you've still got the whole day to get through – how do you cope?

You have less than five minutes *Recharge your own battery.* Go to the toilet / your car / any uninterrupted space you can find and close your eyes to focus on your breath. Set a timer if you are in work – even two to three minutes of focusing on your breathing can provide an energising reset.

You have five to ten minutes *Move.* Ideally a walk in the park would be perfect but if that isn't possible, five to ten minutes around the office, car park, campus, wherever you are.

You have twenty minutes *Nap.* This might be a working from home option only but find a dark space, set a timer, lie down with a little blanket or a jumper, pop on a sleep mask and have a nap. Absolute heaven.

Twenty minutes is the maximum I'd recommend to ensure you feel restored rather than drowsy or jet-lagged on waking.

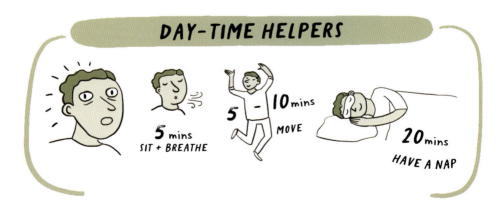

DAY-TIME HELPERS

5 mins
SIT + BREATHE

5 – 10 mins
MOVE

20 mins
HAVE A NAP

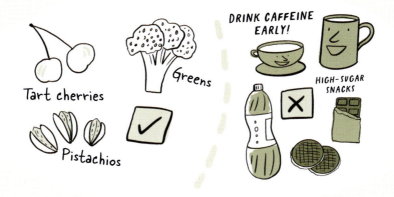

Food and sleep

Caffeine and sugar are stimulants. Knowing that caffeine has a half-life of up to eight hours means that that mid-afternoon vente cappuccino might be lurking in your cells making it harder to fall asleep at bedtime. Similarly, pre-bed snacks that are sugary or high in refined carbohydrate (chocolate biscuits, I'm talking to you) may also make it harder to switch off as the sugar takes a joy ride through your body.

Here are three things to add to your shopping list to help you on your way to the land of nod:

Tart cherries These fruits and their juices can increase our natural melatonin production, as well as the sleep-inducing neurotransmitter tryptophan

Greens Deep-green coloured veg are rich in calcium and magnesium, which are sleep essentials

Pistachios Perfect for an evening snack, these nuts are another rich source of natural melatonin, as well as healthy fats important for serotonin release

Sleep school: when to bring in the experts

Sleep medicine is a speciality of medicine like neurology, dermatology and orthopaedics. That is because there are diseases that are related to sleeping that can be managed and treated.

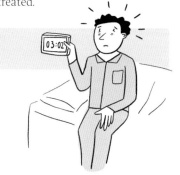

Physical signs that you need more help:

A partner noticing your breathing is pausing or causing you to choke overnight

Sleeping seven to eight hours at night and still feeling exhausted

Persistent night terrors or sleepwalking

When nothing you've tried is working

The difference between sleep and rest

In my first proper GP job, the practice I worked in was about fifteen minutes' drive from my flat. After a full morning surgery followed by patient phone calls and a couple of GP visits, I got into the routine of driving home for lunch. In the middle of the thirty-minute round trip, I'd be left with ten minutes or less to eat my lunch and spend time with my favourite lunchtime date, Peter Andre. There was something unknowingly therapeutic about watching him choosing curtains and calling his agent repeatedly to push for bookings. If something happened and I couldn't follow my lunchtime routine, even though I'd avoided the panic of getting back to the surgery on time, I'd often find myself more tired and stressed about the afternoon ahead.

Taking periods of scheduled rest throughout the day helps with increasing energy and improving problem-solving skills. Research, done as recently as the 1990s, has looked at brain activity in these 'down times' and found that, much like sleep, our brains are active during these times. Just in very different ways.

Functional MRI scans, which map the function of the brain of people who are lying at rest, reveal that even when breathing is accounted for, there remain signs of brain activity that researchers were not expecting to find. Researchers surmised that when you are staring into space, actively doing nothing, your brain is using almost as much energy as when you are solving complex maths problems.

While the energy consumption of the 'doing nothing brain' is similar to the 'busy at work brain', the circuits and connections in these two different states are different.

This has been shown beautifully by studying brain function in action when we read. When we are engrossed in the story, we are using thinking brains, and yet as we dawdle over turning the page, or lose focus as we remember we forgot to put the bin out, our brain moves seamlessly into our downtime state known as the default mode network (DMN).

It might feel frustrating if you are trying to keep track of a plot and you keep losing focus so easily (you might already have done it as you read this page) but there are brain benefits to prioritising regular periods in this downtime state.

When studying this downtime state in children, researchers have found that those with the most active and connected brains here score better in attention, memory, thinking and reading. They also were more empathic.

While I thought I was filling my brain with nonsensical reality TV, I was actually enhancing my ability to pay attention and perhaps even care for my patients in the afternoon surgery.

How to tap into your downtime settings

Allow your mind to wander – by letting your thoughts merrily roll along you enhance your connections within your default network. This improves creativity and wellbeing.

Ageing and life stresses can alter the structure of these networks. BUT we can always activate and improve them by turning our to-do list off for a few minutes and letting our thoughts meander.

Just don't tell your phone about it.

Social media scrolling isn't the same as mind-wandering. Even having your phone near you can impact your creativity and focus. To rest effectively, we need to turn our phones off or at least lock them in a box while we allow our minds time to truly wander uninterrupted.

Up your rest ratio

Schedule We won't rest by accident; we have to make it happen.

Walk One of the few times where doing two things at once is a good idea.

Sleep Converse to what you might think, the better we sleep, the easier it is for us to switch off when we decide to during the day.

Down tools If you don't plan for it, your brain will remind you it needs downtime. When you start to feel your concentration is going and your ideas and focus are dwindling, down tools and take a few minutes off. Research has shown that even looking at a few key positive memory-inducing images on your phone can provide that microbreak you need to help you reset when you are ready. (Note: this is focused phone time with a purpose, as opposed to mindless scrolling!)

We are regularly competing in the Busy Olympics, even if we haven't signed up for a single race. Even hobbies have become side hustles and family day trips are a source of stress.

Our brains remain at the core of who we are and a huge source of our energy consumption. When you feel tired or irritable for no obvious reason, it's worth considering how many brain-caring habits you've been able to prioritise recently. Taking time to rest, scheduling naps when you can, and prioritising sleep are an excellent place to start.

'HOW BEAUTIFUL IT IS DO NOTHING AND THEN TO REST AFTERWARDS.'
— Spanish proverb.

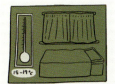
A cool, dark bedroom

SLEEP BASICS

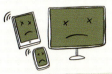
Avoid all screens
1–2hrs before bed

Keep me away from your bed!

DECAF FROM 2 p.m.

Avoid alcohol and large amounts of other liquids close to bed

MORE HELP WITH SLEEP

SET A SLEEP TIME

& WORK BACKWORDS

WIND DOWN BEFORE BEDTIME

KEEP TO A ROUTINE

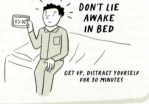
DON'T LIE AWAKE IN BED

Have a beside notebook
MY WORRIES

& use a sleepmask

GET UP, DISTRACT YOURSELF FOR 30 MINUTES

DAY-TIME HELPERS

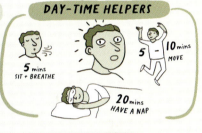
5 mins SIT + BREATHE

5 – 10 mins MOVE

20 mins HAVE A NAP

FOOD AND SLEEP

Tart cherries

Greens

Pistachios

DRINK CAFFEINE EARLY!

HIGH-SUGAR SNACKS

REMEMBER TO...

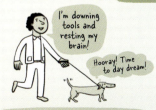
I'm downing tools and resting my brain!

Hooray! Time to day dream!

Take time to rest

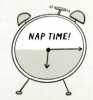
NAP TIME!

Schedule naps if you can

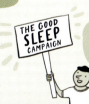
THE GOOD SLEEP CAMPAIGN

But I accept I won't always sleep well!

Prioritse sleep

WRITE, SING, DRAW

Creativity is a way of seeing and doing things differently. Being creative *may* result in a tangible outcome but it is the *process* of creation that brings the most benefits to our brain. It's the doing that matters as opposed to what you have to show for it as a result.

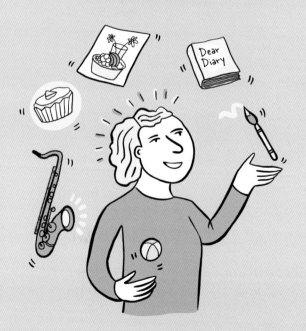

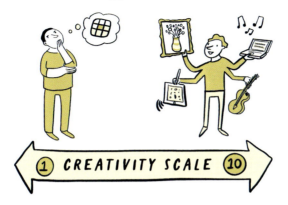

The more creative habits we invest time in, and the more time we spend encouraging creative thinking, the easier this becomes for us and the more our brain benefits.

Robert was a patient whom I'd seen only on a sore-throat-and-occasional-skin-rash-type basis. He was middle-aged in every conventional way, down to his slightly hunched stature, an attempt to obscure his gently expanding mid-region. During one appointment, he pulled out a notebook to write down a website I'd given him and there was the most incredible sketch of an elderly man tucked into the front.

When I asked him about it, he blushed uncharacteristically, seemingly embarrassed that his security-guard cover had been blown. He proceeded to show me a portfolio of art he had drawn of his friends and family over the years on his phone.

When I highlighted how talented he was as an artist, he became flustered and repeatedly eschewed any praise.

Robert, this chapter is for you – and everyone else who gave up drawing / singing / writing / dancing because of 'I'm never going to be good enough at it so what's the point?' syndrome.

WHAT WE THINK CREATIVITY IS: Performing

WHAT CREATIVITY ACTUALLY IS: Activating thought processes that encourage brain cells to connect and function in new ways.

How creative are you?

If I said, let's get creative, what picture pops into your mind? Your four-year-old self with paints and play dough? The creators on social media looking down the barrel of a lens showing you their breakfast? Or maybe it's a theatre-style picture of a stage and costumes and catchy melodies. Perhaps it's not an image at all. It may be a feeling. One that says, *'Nope, I'm not the creative type, I can skip this one.'*

Please don't skip this.

Whether you think you are a creative type or not, this chapter will explain why creativity is about a lot more than a production or a painting.

In its simplest terms, being creative is about being open to self expression – to others or just for yourself. The home of our creative selves is within our brains and remember, our brains are built for survival – to create and make believe is to live.

It's not just in our brains, it's our genes too

Signs of creative talents appeared in our ancestors over three million years ago. But it was 50,000 years ago that the human creative train began to really take off. Statues of imaginary creatures, ornaments and bone flutes all date back to this time.

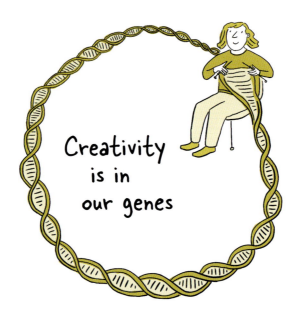

Creativity is in our genes

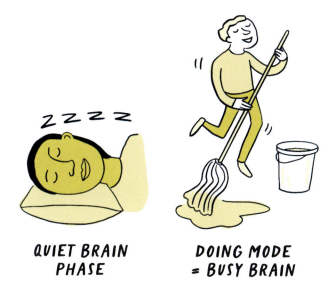

QUIET BRAIN
PHASE

DOING MODE
= BUSY BRAIN

Where do creative ideas come from?

Our ancestors considered creative ability and outputs to be the work of gods, goddesses and spirits, but we have more evidence now that really, it comes from our minds. (Although I think there is still some sort of spirit that helps you sing like a Broadway star or dance like Beyoncé.) In one study, scientists gave participants the challenge of making up a story, then observed the participants' brain wave activity during the process and found two different systems hard at work.

Quiet brain phase, aka inspiration phase

When the story ideas where just part of thoughts and musing, brain wave activity reflected a relaxed state of mind, at times mirroring the levels of brain activity seen in some phases of sleep, dreaming or rest.

Which is why if you are struggling with your next plot point or how to move forward in a dilemma at work, a nap or at least a rest might be a good idea.

Researchers theorised that the subconscious mind was in full flow during this creative thinking phase, rather than the busy mind with all the to-dos and don'ts and worries of every day.

Doing mode, aka busy brain

When participants were asked to actively work on their story ideas, brain wave activity shifted to a busier, but still co-ordinated pattern of activity reflecting conscious and active thoughts.

Thanks to our brain helping us move between subconscious and conscious mind states, we all have the ability to generate and act on these creative ideas but why does this come more easily to some than others? In the same experiment, researchers saw that participants who exhibited the biggest difference in brain activity between these two stages were found to have the most creative ideas. This gave rise to the thinking that the ability of the brain to move between these two channels of creativity may influence whether we are dreamers or dream makers.

What is stopping us creating?

Children draw with no thought of what their picture will look like. They may not even know what it is going to be or why they are doing it. There is a moment, however, when we start to look at each other's pictures. Then one day we will look and decide *'mine is not as good as theirs'.* When we start comparing the outcomes of our creative efforts as older children and teenagers, and we listen to that voice, those are the moments that we decide we 'aren't very good at it' and just stop. Who wants to keep doing something they know they are not very good at?

We've confused creating with the outcome of our creation.

The benefits from undertaking these types of creative activities are inbuilt in doing them.

The fear

When you watch any TV talent show, you can feel that moment when they know they have two minutes to potentially change their life and the whole audience sits in that blind fear with them.

That isn't what the act of being creative needs to feel like. Unless you choose to put your work out there to the world, creative acts are not for others – they are for you.

There is something about being rejected for a creative endeavour that wounds the ego more than when failing a test or losing a race. Performing or creating something is an expression of ourselves. Hearing that what we have presented isn't good enough hurts. For some, this can push an accelerate button to carry on and create anyway. But for most of us, who don't have ambitions for a creative career, these early experiences can hardwire us to marry together that feeling with the practice of expressing ourselves in this, or any other creative way.

In a very sensible effort to avoid re-experiencing that pain, we stop doing it. Our brain is protecting us from this horrible feeling of rejection. But when we can overcome that, amazing things can happen.

When our kids come home from school with 'artwork', we'd never consider looking at it and going 'well that isn't going to be good enough to sell to strangers' and put it straight in the bin. Yet as adults, we do this to ourselves without even thinking about it.

We shut down our creativity based on the fact that the person who sat next to us in art in primary school drew a better fruit bowl than we did. Or a music teacher told us to just mouth the words in choir.

This is why our brains cannot always be trusted.

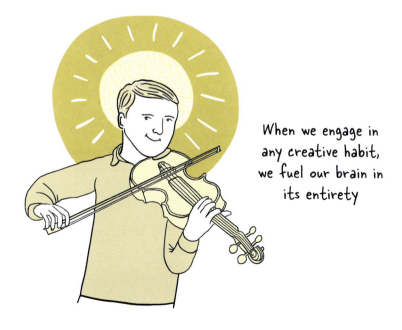

When we engage in any creative habit, we fuel our brain in its entirety

Left brain vs right brain

Historically we talked about left brain vs right brain and equated the right side of the brain with expressive creativity and the left side with being practical and more analytical in thinking and behaviours. Our interest and ability in topics were determined by how dominant each side of the brain was. That is old news. When we engage in any form of creative habit, we fuel our brain in its entirety.

While there may be only a few of us who have the innate talent of a world-class musician, every artist of this level will tell you the same thing: they give hours of dedication to perfecting their craft.

Some may be born with a jaw-dropping ability to create, but it is the time given to the doing that makes them the household names we hold is such high esteem.

Because of the brains' innate ability to change and alter throughout a lifetime we can always help ourselves become more creative.

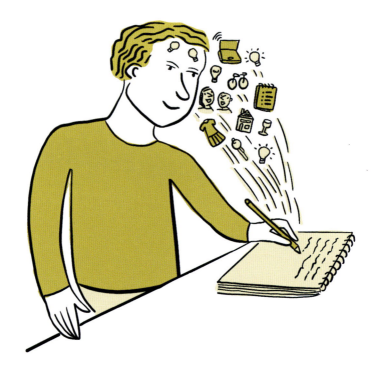

Start by mentally decluttering

Regardless of whether it looks like a tick box to-do list or your thought dump of the day, writing down what is on your mind is an excellent way to clear space for other types of thinking. The act of expunging these thoughts into a tangible form can stop your mind going down into a rabbit hole that it can never come out of.

Writing about ourselves: Reduces stress by creating a distance between what has happened and how we think about it. This helps us process confusing or difficult events that have happened and removes whatever it is from the forefront of our minds to help us gain perspective.

Writing about others: Helps us make sense of relationships around us, and can create a positive memory bank of experiences for our future. It also distracts us from our current challenges.

To-do and ta-dah

My life as a clinical doctor revolved around my to-do list but I learnt early on to always put two things on it that I had already done. This tricked my mind into thinking 'at least I've got a few things done' vs 'I will never get home tonight'. Simple but effective.

A less-used – but equally important list is the To-Don't

- I will not silently fume when my colleague uses my milk for their tea. Instead, I will make a milk buying rota and circulate it.
- I will not read the class Whatsapp before bed tonight
- I will not buy more biscuits 'just in case' there is an apocalypse

To think creatively in life, we can use everyday activities as source material. Every time you think your way out or around a problem, you are engaging a form of creative thinking.

Set the scene for creativity

Being creative is brain fuel – the opportunities for this are like drinking water or eating your greens. Make time for it. The fuel for this is all around us. Think of the sights and sounds going on around you as the opening scene in a film and let your mind imagine what comes next. But make sure to minimise unwanted distractions.

Put your phone on aeroplane mode

As well as your brain telling you that you're not the creative type, that thing in your pocket is the perfect distraction from any sort of creative practice. Looking at other people's creativity on social media doesn't count.

Choose your own soundtrack

When you turn the radio on in the car or put the TV on at home, these noises become the soundtrack to your time. Choose your soundtrack, maybe silence, or songs or music that makes you feel a certain way. When we are relaxed and know what is coming, we can think more clearly.

Slow down

Like every cable in your house, connections between brain cells are insulated. While good insulation is thought to be a key marker of a healthy brain, when it comes to being creative there is (of course) a different point of view to consider.

Studies into the brains of people who are more creative have shown that wiring in some parts of the brain is slower, so could it be those thinking processes mean we don't have time to listen to our inner critic and close down our own creative thoughts before they have even got off our own starting block.

But brain cells use more than wiring to communicate; hormones and chemical neurotransmitters also make a difference. Specifically, noradrenaline is key. In research studies, when people have been given noradrenaline, this slows down their ability to answer puzzles or complete word games as it prevents communication between wider networks of brain cells.

This might explain why lower levels of noradrenaline and states that support this – such as sleepiness or even stages of depression – have been linked to more creative thinking.

Three Ds to help you build your creativity habit

Daydream

The exact opposite of paying attention is important for us. First, it's fun – how will you even know what you are going to spend your lottery win on if you don't allow your mind to wonder about it?

Sailing off on our own mental boat also helps us disconnect from present stresses and worries, so that when you are back on dry land you are that little bit more prepared to face the storm.

But daydreaming does even more than that. Allowing our minds to wander helps them build new connections and forge thinking paths that weren't there before.

Doodle

Scribbling engages default networks in the brain. It's also been shown to improve recall from lists by almost a third. And it's fun. Big companies such as Apple, Ford and Disney encourage their employees to doodle. Those guys know what they are doing.

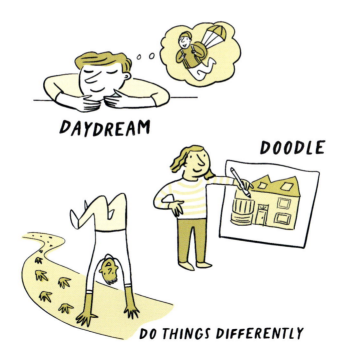

DAYDREAM

DOODLE

DO THINGS DIFFERENTLY

Do things differently

In lockdown, I, probably like you, walked the same pavement at the same time of day for weeks. I saw the same people, walking their same dogs and heard the same eerie silence from the road. About five weeks in, my son said, 'can't we just explore in the field behind our house instead?' It hadn't even crossed my mind. Without realising it, my son was suggesting we try out being *flaneurs* instead of plodding our well-worn path. Translating from the French, this means to wander, with no destination in mind, observing society. When we make even small changes, our problem solving and thinking skills can be given a new lease of life which improves our creativity pathways.

Undercover creativity (you are doing this already)

Our daily word puzzle, game night with our nearest and dearest or walking through the park on our way home. In these simple activities, we can trigger creative thought patterns as we detach from our complex everyday grown-up lives and allow ourselves to focus elsewhere. Even being fully absorbed in our Friday night movie can provide the mental switch off and downtime that can encourage brain creativity and focus when we next sit down to complete a task.

Cooking

The benefits of being creative, as we know, come primarily from the process as opposed to the outcome. But cooking is a two-for-one. In a matter of minutes, we can be creative and fire up those brain cells, be pleased with the outcome and get a nice buzzy dopamine surge and then we get to eat and feel nourished by what we've made. But it seems for many of us, cooking can put us right in our schoolchild artist mindset. We'd rather watch others do it than even begin to try the process for ourselves. At any point of the day or night we can watch cookery shows or scroll through videos of other people cooking. Yet for over 50 per cent of us, that does not translate to more cooking time. Why? Are we secretly convinced we aren't very good at it so watch the experts instead?

Trying to cook like Gordon Ramsay when you've never made a successful omelette is self-sabotage and reaffirms our brain's safety catch. It will prevent us from eating our uncooked food while confirming the lie that we can't cook.

Instead, start simple and go from there. And keep going.

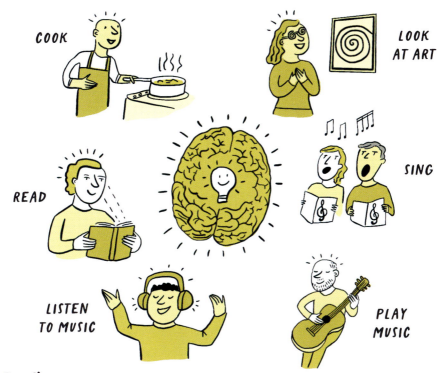

COOK

LOOK AT ART

READ

SING

LISTEN TO MUSIC

PLAY MUSIC

Reading

Shown to encourage empathy, improve mood and encourage brain connections, reading has creative and mood brain benefits falling out on every page. Audiobooks have been shown to have similar benefits.

Singing

Whether you can hold a tune or not does not matter for brain health (although it might matter to your audience).

When we sing, we strengthen our vagus nerve, the nerve that connects our gut, lungs and heart to our brain. The longest nerve in the body, it has a crucial role in mediating our stress responses and how we relax. Singing, or even just humming, is a proven way to improve these connections and this in turn helps our both our relaxation skills and creative processes.

Research with stroke patients found that even though they couldn't speak, they could still sing 'Happy Birthday'. The scientist who discovered this was able to use music-fuelled speech therapy to help these patients regain their ability to speak.

Listening to music

Music – listening to and playing it – lights up our whole brain, from front to back. It is used therapeutically to help children with autism, as a treatment for depression and anxiety, to improve tremor and gait in people with Parkinson's, and as a therapy for even late-stage Alzheimer's dementia patients.

Not only that, music gives all of us another chance at living creatively. We all have our own unique memory playlist that accompanies some of our best and worst moments. Music can change our mood, trigger nostalgia and make us move to a beat. And listening to background music triggers our downtime thinking processes, known as the default mode network (DMN).

Looking at art

Research done by the BBC looked at what happens in our brains when we look at a classical painting. Using EEG sensors, they were able to see how the subjects' brains lit up, or not, depending on what they were looking at and how this was interpreted.

When most participants saw things they recognised, the brain areas reflecting problem solving and conscious thought lit up.

But what was most fascinating from this research is how the responses varied between a group of people looking at the same artwork.

Maybe your primary school fruit bowl painting seen by a different brain would have been viewed as a masterpiece?

Neuroaesthetics

In the same way that sleep, diet and rest have been under the brain research microscope in recent years as we seek to understand how they really impact our brain function, art is currently undergoing this level of study. Neuroaesthetics is about using technology and the latest research tools to understand more about how and why art-filled experiences have such a positive impact on our brains and, consequently, our health.

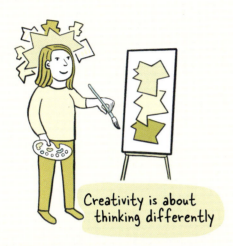

Creativity is about thinking differently

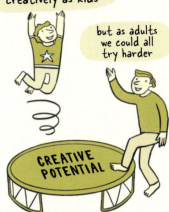

we are at our best creatively as kids

but as adults we could all try harder

CREATIVE POTENTIAL

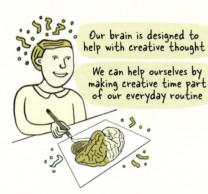

Our brain is designed to help with creative thought

We can help ourselves by making creative time part of our everyday routine

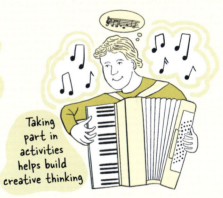

Taking part in activities helps build creative thinking

Doodling, daydreaming, daring to think differently helps our creativity

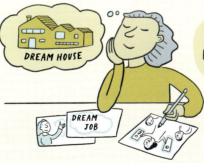

DREAM HOUSE

DREAM JOB

Ignore any negative voices. They aren't real

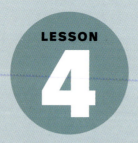

COOK, FEED, NOURISH

Your brain consumes 20 per cent of your energy.
If we can upgrade the fuel we are using for this
energy, we can move from flying economy to
flying first class.

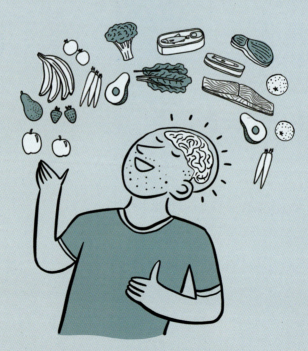

First, let's start with the most important point. With global statistics such as one in ten people going to bed hungry every night, and three billion people unable to afford a nutritious diet, even having a conversation about how and what we eat is a privilege.

If, like me, you are in the position to choose what you buy to cook, then it makes sense that we think about what we are eating and why.

FOOD IS IMPORTANT FOR OUR BRAINS

Research over the last decade has confirmed that what we eat, and how much of it, has a role in the functioning of our brain. We know now that food and nutrition can be used as an adjunctive treatment in mental health conditions such as depression and anxiety. Research done in Australia looked at a group of patients who were suffering from depression and anxiety and randomised them into two groups, one received brain-healthy dietary advice and counselling, the other just received counselling. By the end of the trial the group who had received the food intervention had a 30 per cent reduction in depressive symptoms compared to those who just received counselling. The reduction in anxiety symptoms was also significant and these results have been replicated in other small trials since then.

Perhaps these findings are not surprising. Food, after all, provides an energy source to fuel brain function, has an impact on inflammation and influences microbiome and gut health.

This is the only science lesson in this book. Please don't skip it.

Let's try to consider the scale of what we are talking about.

Your brain is an organ that contains more than eighty billion neurons and has more connections than there are stars in the galaxy. Neurons are just one of type of brain cell that forms the structural foundations of our brain. As well as glial cells to insulate neurons, there are also fibres made by brain cells to further facilitate communication So, we've got an idea of the structural elements, now we need blood supply via blood vessels and chemicals to fly around to help everyone communicate and get along. These chemicals are the neurotransmitters you've probably read about: dopamine, serotonin, adrenaline and endocannabinoids. One more thing to note is the cell receptors that collect the neurotransmitters on the surface of the cell to help the message land (literally). There is a lot going on up top and when you realise this, it makes more sense why nourishment is so important. Our brains, despite being only 2 per cent of our body weight, consume 20 per cent of everything we eat.

Your brain is a growth machine

Up until the mid-1990s, the understanding was that the brain cells we had were ours for life to enjoy/destroy as we chose.

But then, like so much in science, things pivoted when it was discovered that our brain cells are the play dough of cells that can be built, grown and changed throughout our lives.

When we read about a ninety-year-old weightlifting or a retiree starting a new business, this is why.

If we hear a relative say, *I'm old – there's nothing more I can do about it now*', feel free to tell them (gently) that just isn't true.

On a cellular level, changes can be made at any stage of life. If we fuel ourselves in the best way we can, this gives us not only the best chance of having healthier cells to make these changes with but also the most resilient mindset to want and be able to make them.

A diet rich in omega 3s (see box below) and brain healthy nutrients can help with learning, mood and memory.

Nutrients that support brain health

Omega 3 fatty acids – help maintain healthy glial cells, fight inflammation

Magnesium – building blocks for brain cells and help create those important neurotransmitters

B vitamins – a personal favourite of mine, b vitamins help with conducting nerve impulses, as well as reducing inflammation

Iron – mood-regulating neurotransmitters and helps carry oxygen to your brain via blood flow

Vitamin C – antioxidant that keeps brain cells healthy, a sidekick in many biochemical reactions in the brain

Brain-derived neurotrophic factor (BDNF) – our brain cell fairy dust

There may be a lexicon and series of hashtags around brain-impacting chemicals such as serotonin and dopamine, but the less cool cousin of these guys is BDNF – brain-derived neurotrophic factor. It's a protein (building block) that exists only within our brain and associated tissue to help brain cells grow and protect them from evil forces such as stress and toxins. Scientists report when you sprinkle a little BDNF on brain cells in a lab setting you can see them change right there in front of you.

Think of it as our brain cell fairy dust.

The bad news is that BDNF production naturally decreases with age. The good news is we can influence our natural production of BDNF by what we eat.

Our bodies' defences

Next up, we need to talk about inflammation. You might have heard of it as the body's natural response to, say, an injury or an open wound. Our body's defence systems produce this inflammatory response to help us heal. But what we've now discovered is that many aspects of modern life are actually pro-inflammatory.

What? But life's not an injury.

Well, not like a gaping wound or a sprained ankle. However, the chemical responses induced in our cells from chronic stress, smoking, environmental toxins and obesity also have a similar effect over time. It can be hard to remove chronic stresses and eliminate environmental toxins, but while we are working on those, what we eat can help reduce this inflammatory load and strengthen our cells against it.

What happens in your brain when you eat

When you start to eat, nerve cells in your stomach fire up to your brain. At the same time, signals are despatched from your brain to your gut via hormones in the blood stream. These register that we are eating, but take a little bit longer than the nerve-cell signals that go from your stomach. This means that your brain begins to digest food before you even eat it. In anticipation of eating your stomach secretes acid and insulin release begins.

If you think food tastes better when you are hungry you are right, your taste buds are more sensitive the hungrier you are. Each mouthful satisfies that hunger so it's less tasty by the end than it is in the beginning BUT if you switch to something else on your plate, the taste buds reset.

BDNF helpers (to help you make your own brain fairy dust)

Researchers in Spain looked at three groups to understand more about specific foods and if they impacted BDNF levels over four years, The groups were:

1 People on a low-fat diet

2 People following a Mediterranean diet + extra olive oil

3 People following a Mediterranean diet + extra nuts.

Those in group 3 were found to have the highest levels of BDNF.

So certain foods really can help us make more BDNF, specifically:

Berries – rich in antioxidants

Wild-form seafoods – higher dietary intake of brain-power-player omega 3 fatty acids

Pumpkin seeds – support the brain-friendly mineral zinc

Nuts (unsalted) – high in fibre and unsaturated fats.

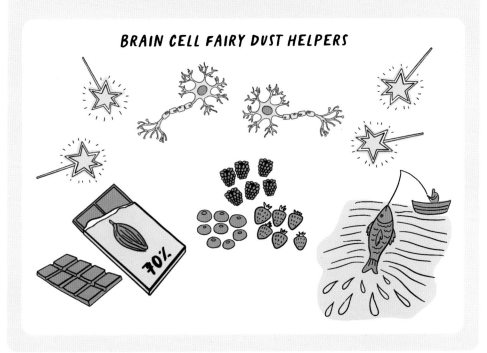

BRAIN CELL FAIRY DUST HELPERS

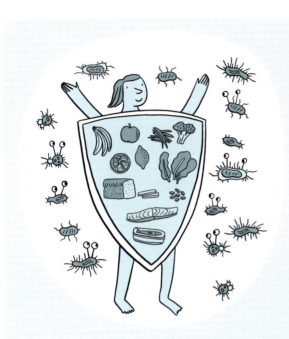

Inflammation shields

Antioxidants – lots of fruit and veg

Omega 3-rich foods – healthy fats to support your brain.

Fibre – gut friendly, helps your feel full and reduces snacking tendencies

It's not all about hunger

Certain tastes are hardwired as being delicious. While Nora Ephron's novel *Heartburn* reminds us of the mood-enhancing power of mashed potatoes, for many of us sadness leads us to sweet treats. These foods trigger brain-chemical feedback loops meaning you want more of the pleasurable feeling so you eat more of these foods regardless of whether you are hungry for any of them. That's why those giant bags of sweets you get in the cinema or take on a road trip give our brain a real challenge.

On the other hand, stress can impact appetite centres in your brain meaning you go off your food. But once the acute stress has passed, or during chronic stress, this can be reversed so your appetite increases instead.

And that's where comfort food steps in. If certain food makes us feel more comfortable with whatever is going on around us, we will want more of it. We pick this up early in life, and from there end up using eating to numb emotional pain.

The S-word

Sugar is a modern day health problem. Glucose is the main source of fuel for our brain. And yes, glucose is sugar. So why is it, then, that sugar in our diet has been shown to be bad for our brain health?

In studies of people with diabetes, both type one and type two, where the key issue is that the body cannot produce or use insulin efficiently to break down sugars, the brain's ability to function was impacted by high blood glucose levels. On top of this, accelerated ageing and small vessel disease were also seen, which further jeopardises healthy brain cell function.

Routines and Rituals

My patient, Eileen, would bring a packet of biscuits to every appointment for me to share out at the teabreak. Every time, I said thank you, there really was no need. She told me her mother had always done it and her sister did too. They took biscuits to the optician, the hospital and even the vet.

We all have routines and quirks around food, snacks and mealtimes. These may be cultural, familiar or just personal habit. The crisps on the way home, the biscuits before bed, road trip sweets – most of us know this isn't driven by hunger, it's more about choices and behaviours rather than nourishment and nutrition. Maybe you have to add butter to your mash, even when it's already in there. From your coffee order and mug you use for your tea in the morning, being aware of your rituals and why you do them can be helpful.

Sugar can also alter how our brain chemicals work – part of the reason that chocolate muffin tastes so good is because feel-good dopamine gets a big kick out of sugar which motivates us to look for this rush again. How do we do this? We eat more chocolate.

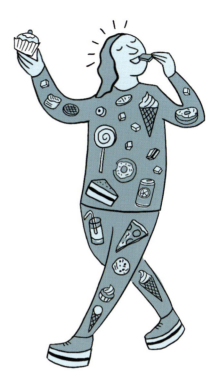

The sugar we know about in the cake that we decide to eat is one thing. But the bigger issue is the sugar and artificial sweeteners that are lurking in most tins and packs in our cupboard. In addition, we've got the breakdown of delicious, refined carbohydrates from bagels or pasta into starch which essentially become a form of sugar in our bodies. From breakfast cereals and toast and jam, to sandwiches and chocolate, to pizza and ice cream – that's a lot of sugar that is just waiting get into our body and mind.

One of my favourite meals is a delicious pizza so let me be clear, I know this is a complicated issue. But what we need to understand, to help us make healthier choices throughout our lives if we can, is that we can manage all of this better if we just think about it a little bit more.

A couple of slices of pizza on a Friday isn't going to be the thing that gives you diabetes when you are middle-aged, neither is having an ice cream when the sun begins to peek through. (Is there anything better than that first cone of summer?)

The goal is to look at what we are eating on a regular basis and know that for the most part, we are choosing nutrient-rich minimally processed foods to fill our plates and fuel our brains.

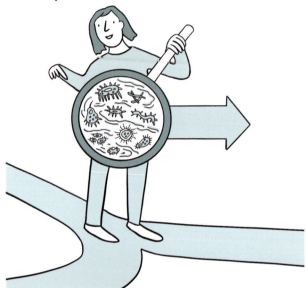

My microbiome is in charge!

Gut–brain connection

It's clear, then, that our brain has an interest in eating that moves beyond nutrition, but whatever it encourages us to put in our bodies will eventually be absorbed, and that's where the gut comes in. The gut is a vast network of cells that contain most of your immune system and also do a fair bit of hormone creation. And on top of them there is the layer of organisms that make up our microbiome.

Our microbiome is the humungous (technical term) mass of bacteria and other bugs that live in our gut. The human body contains roughly thirty trillion human cells and about thirty-eight trillion bacteria, and this band of bugs has the capability to influence many aspects of our health. Bacteria are critical to our immune response to any form of assault (Covid, I'm looking at you) and, of course, are hugely personal.

Our gut is in a fully co-dependent relationship with our brain. Like all long-term relationships, things ebb and flow over the years but overall, it's usually pretty good. When our guts are unhappy (stress, that dodgy chicken burger) our brain knows about it.

But I don't have to tell you that. You know that sick feeling you get when you are called in to see your boss, that excited flutter on a second date with The One and the last-minute run to the toilet before any big moment.

Eating for your gut

Don't worry, I'm going to keep this bit simple. While there is a lot in the media about eating to support your gut health, we can all do one thing that will help: eat more fibre.

Fibre is the secret sauce. It's a **prebiotic**, providing sustenance for healthy gut bacteria. An important way that eating fibre works to support our microbiome is via the release of a breakdown product: short chain fatty acids (SCFAs). These SCFAs are released within our gut as the bacteria chomp on the fibre we've consumed. Animal studies have shown that low levels of SCFAs are associated with increased anxiety and depression. Studies are ongoing to understand further if higher SCFA levels could have the opposite effect. The SCFA butyrate has been shown to reduce inflammation, specifically in conditions such as inflammatory bowel disease.

Fibre has a **low glycaemic index**, which allows for the steady increase of blood sugar rather than a rollercoaster of sugar highs and crashes. Fewer blood sugar spikes are better for our metabolism and can help with blood-pressure control. High blood

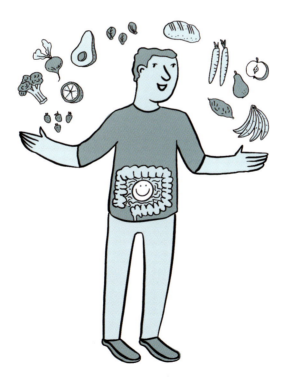

pressure is a key modifiable risk factor for Alzheimer's disease. By reducing cravings and urges to eat sweet foods, better blood glucose control even helps our sleep.

Our gut bacteria play an integral role in formation of important neurotransmitters including serotonin, which is just one of the reasons there is research into how improving our gut metabolism and eating to support a healthy microbiome can improve mental health.

We've covered a lot here, and the reason is that eating, nutrition and diets are probably some of the most complex areas of health and human behaviours because so many factors influence what ends up on our plates, in our mouths, and then how it's absorbed by our gut and finally impacts our brain.

Check list

There is always a lot of noise and mixed messages when it comes to food and nutrition. Everyone is an expert and I find that confusing and exhausting.

Let's keep it simple so we can devote our energy to using the fuel we are consuming, rather than wasting it on worrying if we're eating the 'right' things.

Increase:	Decrease:
Nutrient rich food – ask yourself: 'What nutritional fuel is on my plate?'	Sugar (you know why)
Home-cooked meals	Processed and prepackaged foods when you can
Healthy fats and antioxidant intake (fish, eggs, nuts, greens, berries)	
Fibre – happy gut, happy brain.	

ENJOY WHAT YOU EAT AND WHO YOU EAT IT WITH.

PAY ATTENTION TO YOUR THOUGHTS AND BEHAVIOURS ABOUT FOOD AND HOW YOU FEEL AFTER YOU EAT.

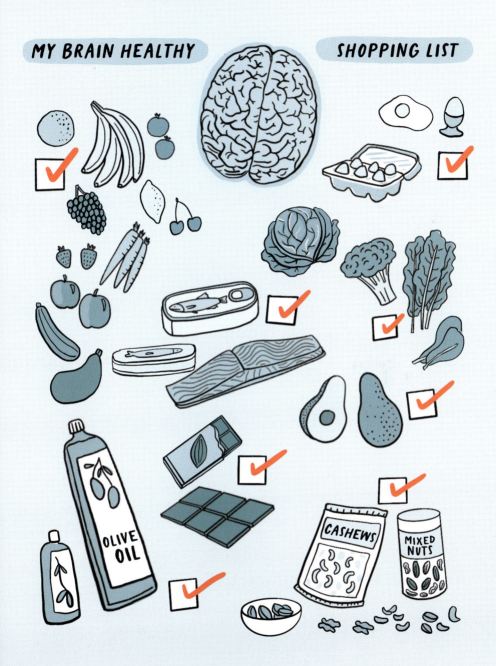

MY BRAIN HEALTHY   SHOPPING LIST

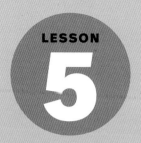

LESSON 5

QUIT, RUN, HIDE

ANYTHING CAUSING YOU STRESS AT THE MOMENT?

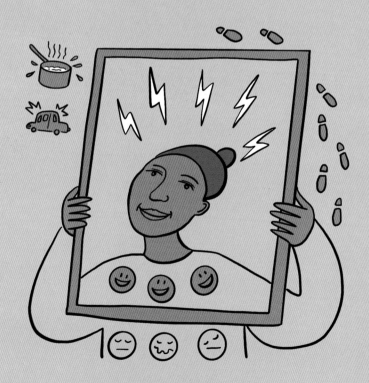

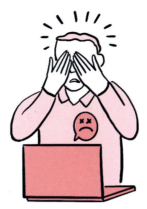

Let's reframe how our brain deals with stress

Let's be clear. Stress is an essential part of life. It keeps us awake, safe and alive because we are primed to react to potential stresses for survival. This stress – the acute stress reaction, known as 'fight or flight', is the type of stress we aren't usually aware of until it kicks in. It's just there, ready to leap into action when a threat is detected.

That stress can still feel horrible as we take dramatic lifesaving action. But any aftermath is usually quickly forgotten as we visualise the likely alternative ending if our brain had not detected that danger, resulting in our bodies' red-light warning system kicking in.

Acute danger rarely occurs in slow motion. Thankfully, stress changes how our cells function. Firing of adrenaline and other neurotransmitters speeds up the chemical impulses that happen within our cells. This is designed to be transient and limited to the threatening event. Once we've dodged the hopefully metaphorical bullet, these chemicals stand down and all our bodily processes return to a neutral stance

This stress is the security alarm of our brain that we don't even have to consciously set.

But *that* stress isn't the one we need to talk about.

It's all the other stress that is the problem.

The feeling when *that* name appears on our phone. Another email from *that* boss that makes us want to cry. The sight of the figure on the bottom of our credit card bill that narrows our field of vision. Then there are all the other things that we can't even name that shift our internal barometer subtly but just far enough that we don't reset. How can we stop *that* stuff from turning up the dial on our stress settings?

Low-level stress and our brains

A stressed brain doesn't know if it's coming or going. It won't pick the healthy choice for anything – from who to date to what to buy for lunch. Because as amazing as our brains are, they can't tell the difference between the things causing the stress in our lives. They are there to keep us alive, not to help us choose low-sugar and organic over fries and a milkshake.

Our brains react to the cellular changes that occur when the stress response sets in. While they will detect if it's not a code red situation, they cannot determine much more than that. When these low-level, slow-burning stress responses occur over days, weeks, even years, we now have a brain functioning on permanent amber light. Consequently, without even realising, we are constantly bracing for impact and about to grab onto whatever there is to try to soften the blow.

Another glass of wine? *Absolutely!*

Another episode of the latest binge-worthy TV show or go to bed early?

You know where this is going.

I know *I* do.

Reframe

We cannot destress our lives; instead let's look at how we can reframe situations and stressors to be able to deal with all those issues better. In Chapter one I talked about my Stop, Look, Listen method (see pages 8–17) and that can be really helpful here to find out what's really bothering you. From there, you have the choice to either make positive changes or continue to tread down well-worn paths.

Just feel it

It helps to start by acknowledging what is going on for you so that you can respect how you feel. By doing this, you don't dilute your empathy or compassion for people with 'bigger' problems. In fact, you can often offer more of yourself to them and their needs by honouring your own situation first. Give yourself time and grace and, crucially, ask for help if you need it.

Well-worn paths than can be unhelpful

When you get used to listening to yourself, validating your feelings and honouring what's happening for you, you'll start noticing pieces of advice that are a lot less helpful than people intend them to be.

It could be worse . . .

'It could be worse, at least it isn't cancer.'

I was told this and, and told myself this, many times when I was trying to come to terms with having MS.

Is comparing bad stuff the way we should reframe our stress?

NO!

In the same way our brain can't determine the cause of our stress and can only act on the impact, the same is true for ourselves.

To be able to manage stresses better we have to acknowledge them not dismiss them into 'it could be worse' fog.

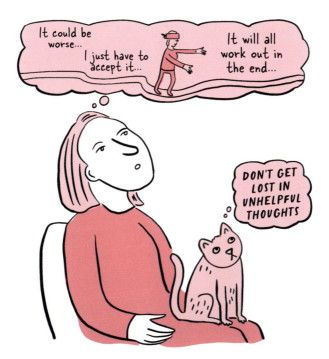

'It will all work out in the end'

This might sound harsh, as of course things will work out in some capacity, but the real question is: *'At what cost?'*

Doing nothing in the face of chronic stress is akin to leaving the bath tap dripping with the plug in. It might take ages to overflow, but when it does, the damage can be substantial. And while the tap has been dripping, you've been paying more than you should have been for water, too.

Sometimes we just have to face up to difficult situations. Confronting the source of why we feel the way we do is never easy. Once we've looked inwards and determined what the issue is, there are often external factors that need addressing.

It's just how it is – I just have to accept it

Do you? What would happen if you spoke up?

Our brains want to keep us safe, and for them it is very definitely a case of 'better the devil you know'. An unhappy situation that is known and 'under control' is much more appealing to our brains than the great unknown. But the potential for greater happiness is in taking the leap.

Making changes

When you realise that it's time to shift or change things up, it can sometimes feel like a fight against your brain. Everything in you might be screaming to return to the safety of the known, so you'll need tools and support to make things different.

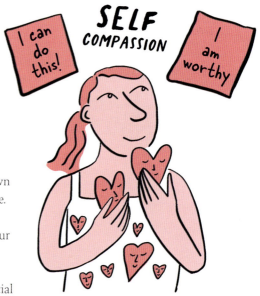

Self-compassion

Recognise that it is hard and be your own cheerleader as you take on this challenge. You may feel like the only one on your side speaking up, so you need to sing your own chant here (even if it's just in your head). And don't be afraid to find other people who will support you. We are social animals and get enormous strength and resilience from others. Affirmations on a sticky note or a little note by your bed can also be really useful here, but keep them simple, for example 'I am kind' 'I am worthy' 'I can do this'.

Accept it will be hard
Challenging situations are rarely a one and done. It's not an episode of your favourite TV drama that will be resolved in twenty-eight minutes. These things take time, continued self-bravery and courage before there is resolution.

Watch your language
Our brain is constantly listening to our thoughts and reinforces what these are. When things are tough, it can be easy to turn the blame on yourself and have a self-narrative of negativity. This will almost certainly happen when you find yourself in a situation of conflict. Try changing 'I'm an idiot' to 'I'm OK'. In time, replace 'I'm OK' with 'I'm good'. Eventually, you will be able to congratulate yourself that you've done a really hard thing that took guts and bravery. No one else might say it to you so I will:

WELL DONE, YOU'VE DONE AN AMAZINGLY HARD THING THAT SHOWED YOUR COURAGE, STRENGTH AND GRACE.

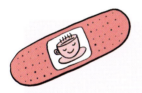

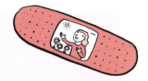

Sticking Plasters

When it all feels too much, these quick fixes can really help:

Tea – calming benefits of L-theanine provide stress relief in a cup

Rest – even a few minutes of intentional rest reduces cortisol

Walk outside – improves brain blood flow and offers soothing benefits of nature

Channel change – distract yourself with something that will bring a positive outcome. Cook, write a card to a friend or visit a museum.

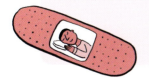

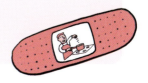

Kintsugi – we are stronger in the broken places

Where you end up may not be where you wanted or planned to be.

Even if you don't get what you thought you wanted, by facing up to what has caused you so much stress you have done something amazing. Even if it feels horrible now, you will be different and stronger for it eventually.

Trust me, I'm a doctor.

Waves vs ripples

It would be great if stresses came like waves and one had to crash before the next one could come.

Sadly, life is not like that.

How often have you experienced that sense of 'if one more thing happens, I am going to lose it'. And then it does?

These events may feel like ripples because you are already feeling the impact of the stone being dropped in the water. That stressed brain is already operational so the next thing and the one after just gradually feel bigger and eventually can feel all-consuming and unsurmountable.

Even when it feels like ripples, it is actually waves.

Everything will eventually pass, and you will still be you.

Reading about how to deal with it isn't the same as dealing with it

When I was struggling to come to terms with having MS, I sourced information from anywhere I could. Books, documentaries and listening to podcasts about others who had faced chronic illness, struggled with self-doubt in their career or parenting helped.

I took a hugely respected and recommended book about tackling stress on holiday with me and by the pool, as my son slept, I opened the page, highlighter and pencil at the ready and waited patiently for the a-ha moments that were going to mean I'd come home from holiday fixed.

I couldn't get past the first chapter. I read and reread those pages about twenty times on that holiday. Why didn't they make sense? Why wasn't I immediately enlightened and armed with a self-cure tool kit?

Because I had the constant amber stress light on which was running in parallel with the red one. I was anxious, exhausted, burnt out and constantly worried. Even

Hard times cheat sheet

Self-check-in is even more important in times like these. Always have a sense of how you are for yourself.

Ask yourself where there are cracks. Without attending to them, they will deepen and break us open. If we are aware of what is causing them then we can make changes as we go.

When the worst happens – and it will – know that you will be ok. And that even when everyone around you looks like they are swanning through life without a care, everyone faces sad, hard and painful moments.

Everything will feel worse when you aren't tending to the basics.

Prioritise sleep, take a short walk every day.

Limit the junk food, drink more water than you feel like doing and make time for something fun.

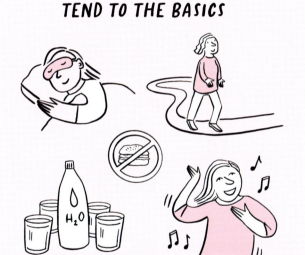

TEND TO THE BASICS

Marian Keyes couldn't provide me comfort or a laugh, let alone a high-brow research scientist with more letters after her name than an alphabet.

Stress can be contagious so don't be surprised if those around you start to appear stressed too. Research undertaken during public speaking showed that cortisol levels in the audience matched the levels of the speaker.

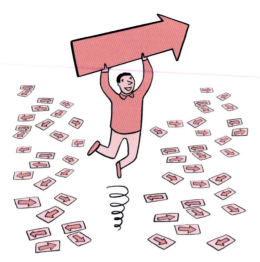

Make 'good-enough' decisions

Decision-making is not only the cause of stress but can also be impacted by feeling stressed. How do we ever know if we are making the right decision? From the big stuff to the everyday, there is no rule book to follow or teacher telling you what is right or wrong. As a result, deciding on big stuff (sometimes small stuff too) can be extremely mentally draining. You are putting your brain through a full workout as it plays out lots of 'what if 'scenarios for you. A decision that is 'good enough' may actually be the answer according to research – *and* less mentally exhausting as you haven't invested so much of yourself into making it.

Celebrating your wins

Decide – from the Latin *decidere* meaning 'cut' and *caedere* 'off'.

Well done you've done it, you have cut off those 17,000 'what if' options that have been weighing you down and chosen one. This is the moment to exhale, move on and celebrate your decisiveness.

Depending on the nature of your decision you might not feel like blowing up the balloons, but having the strength and courage to face into your options, weigh-up choices and settle on a path that you have decided is the right one for you, is always a moment for a round of applause. Unless your decision ends with you bowing on a stage, no one else might actually clap for you, so take time to mark this step for yourself. Even if it's only with an early night (deciding is EXHAUSTING), a walk around the shops or a wee piece of cake; acknowledge your progress and remember that the decision you have made is always the right one.

If you are thinking that's a bit much, remember that creating positive experiences after stressful times can help our brain pull on this resource the next time the stress-ometer starts to rise.

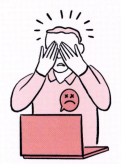

HOW EVERYDAY STRESS MAKES US FEEL IS OFTEN ABOUT OUR REACTIONS

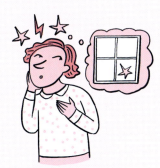

SUPRESSING STUFF DOESN'T MAKE IT GO AWAY

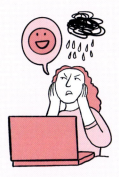

PRETENDING THINGS ARE OK JUST ADDS TO THE STRESS

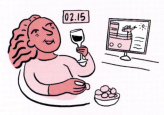

OUR TIRED BRAINS LOOK FOR THE PATH OF LEAST RESISTANCE

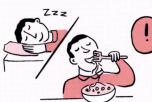

MAKE REST AND GOOD FOOD A PRIORITY

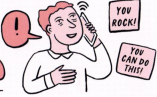

FACE IN, SUPPORT YOURSELF AND ASK FOR HELP

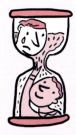

BE PATIENT, THIS ALL TAKES TIME

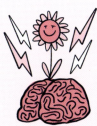

YOUR BRAIN WILL THEN REACT DIFFERENTLY TO PERIODS OF STRESS

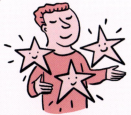

TAKE TIME TO ACKNOWLEDGE AND REWARD YOURSELF

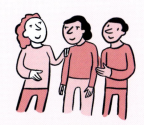

YOU ARE NOT ALONE, PEOPLE WILL SUPPORT YOU

YOU, ME, THEM

As a GP, visiting patients at home was both a privilege and often the most logistically challenging part of the day. Mary was a patient who had regular house calls to review ongoing minor but life-impacting symptoms. Itchy dry skin, a painful fungal toenail and, most commonly, just not feeling herself, though she was always smiling. When I left her one day, she thanked me for visiting, as was her usual lovely way, and then said, 'After the doctor has been, I feel better already. Can you ask the nurse to come tomorrow?'

WHO WE SURROUND OURSELVES WITH AND THE WAY WE CONNECT CAN SHAPE MORE THAN WHAT FILLS OUR DAY.

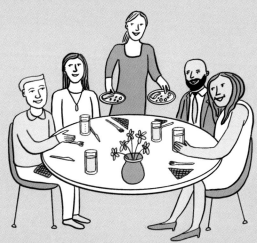

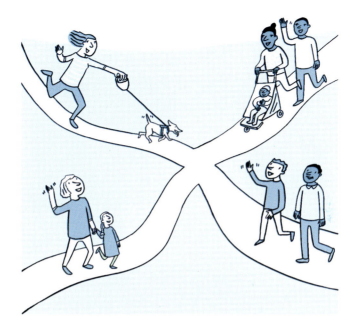

Seeing people in real life is good for us

Our brains are wired for connection so when they see another face, those important positive-impact brain chemicals are released. Dopamine and oxytocin surge through our nervous system and cortisol lowers.

Women are more likely to see trusted friends on a more regular basis than men and some researchers are clear that this is a key reason why women live longer than men.

Three trusted and secure relationships seem to hold the scientific key to the benefit of connections for our health and wellbeing.

The data supports this: for men who have had a stroke and women who have had breast cancer, having regular face-to-face meetings with social connections improved their post-disease outcomes.

We have been built to connect. To form partnerships and communities, and flourish and grow as a result. Our whole lives are designed around connections – from love connections to family roots, to the colleagues we spend eight hours a day with and the friends that move in and out of our lives as the decades roll on.

Our brains support and thrive on these connections. The most 'social' of all the organs, our brain cells wire and fire together to support learning. More than that, when we are deprived of connection, our brains react. Every aspect of our physical and mental health is hardwired to form these life-affirming connections.

Our daytime waking hours are consumed by the people we have around us and the relationships we have with them. From the tiniest interaction at a coffee shop to participating in a team building event at work, there is no avoiding how those around us impact how we feel.

Every single relationship we have in our lives is a two-way street.

Even the relationships we were born or have married into.

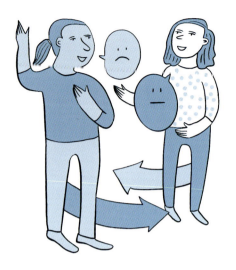

How you are impacts those around you, too

We are so wired and primed to connect to those around us that our brain cells have a reflective capacity to help us do this called 'mirror neurons'. Like Maya Angelou told us, people will never forget how you made them feel and we don't need to look any further for proof of that than Taylor Swift and her Eras tour. She may have broken ticket sales and attendance records but it might be the emotional impact of attending the show that her fans benefit from the most. As well as the avalanches of global positive reviews, some fans even reported post-show amnesia, thought to be a consequence of the intense level of positive emotion experienced from attending the show. As talented as Taylor is, this impact is also due to her audience and the contagious way the smiles of Swifties influenced the mirror neurons of the people around them

Forming relationships

Forming relationships is a cornerstone in our lives. But no one really tells us how to form happy, healthy, balanced connections. As children, we learn from what we see and, sometimes, as parents, we can only offer what we have. We do the best with what we have. But sometimes, actually quite a lot of the time, that can be really really hard.

At work

A challenging dynamic with your boss doesn't have to look like you are in the boardroom of *The Apprentice* to feel horrible. When you work in healthcare, for example, there is a universal common goal which is the wellbeing of the patient you are treating. Even if there are complex dynamics in the healthcare team, we all have the same primary focus. But when I'd listen to my patients with jobs in everything from childcare and local councils to banking, I'd hear tales of the way people are treated and deal with each other in other fields. Personalities, communication styles and target-focused stress often combined into a melting pot of playground behaviours that could have physical and mental health impacting outcomes. While I only ever heard my patients' side of the story, I knew the difficulties people faced in in various work place scenarios could result in the need for time off or ongoing medical support.

As an employee we remain vulnerable at all times as our livelihood remains at stake.

As an employer we carry responsibilities and vulnerabilities of our own.

It is our duty to learn to care for ourselves so we can have the work life we deserve.

You can improve your relationships at work with one thing: *listening*.

Rarely can issues in the workplace be solved immediately and by one person. Often, they require much bigger solutions that may or may not even be feasible. So, although Mary Poppins might not be flying around our offices with her bag of fixits, we can still help each other feel better at work and improve the quality of our work relationships just by listening to each other better. When we listen with both ears open, we reduce loneliness in the workplace, improve social connections and improve feelings of self-esteem on both sides.

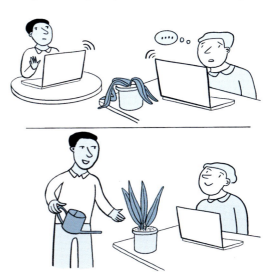

Adult friendships

Some friendships are truly special. We may only have one in a lifetime. We may have new ones at each stage of our lives

But you know that one.

The person you will always smile at when their name pops up on your phone. The one you will spend time with joyfully and in total peace as you talk about nothing and everything.

If you have that in your life, care and nurture that relationship. And tell them how important they are to you. It's easy to be complacent when it comes to friends, we think they will always be there. But they have life and its challenges going on, too. And who doesn't want to be told how much they mean to someone?

On the other hand, friendships do not have to last forever to be important to you. Not continuing to send a Christmas card or acknowledging your kids' birthdays doesn't mean that you have failed or been a bad friend. People come and go from our lives, and just because you met them at six, sixteen or at antenatal class, doesn't mean you need to anchor them into the story of your life forever or place yourself into theirs.

'It would be great to catch up.'

When you get that message or find yourself typing that out, ask yourself do I REALLY want to see this person?

Why haven't I seen them more often?

If you don't know the answers to those questions and can feel nothing but good vibes, then get the doodle poll going.

If you feel a small trickle of uncertainty, listen to that.

Time is precious, so don't waste it trying to recreate something that was fun in high school but doesn't feel that good now.

At home

It was Michelle Obama who introduced me to the concept of good vs bad years in a marriage and it stuck with me as an important way to consider the challenges we can face in long term relationships.

As we age, priorities change and our emotional resources are squeezed, things can feel very different to the nights where you and your partner talked until 3 a.m. about everything and nothing.

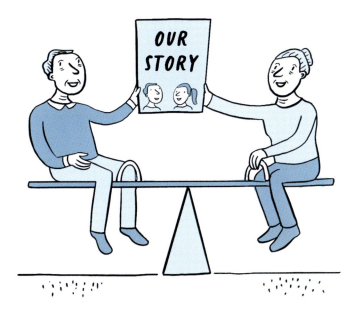

Research supports that being happy in a stable romantic partnership can lead to lower rates of depression, disease and a reduced risk of dementia.

However, we can only give and take with what we have, and that isn't always very much. When both of you have little reserve in the tank at the same time, our relationships can feel off balance.

Our brain can keep us stuck and focused on the immediacy of an argument, or unable to see the way through times of unhappiness.

Self-awareness is at the core of every important relationship you will have. If you are an adult who has been in any form of relationship with another adult, you know how hard it is to get another person to change to your beat. You have to get your footwork in order first.

Feeling lonely vs being alone

Loneliness has been described by the US Surgeon General as 'the most common condition' he saw patients suffer with. Described as an epidemic in the US, post pandemic statistics in the UK state that up 50 per cent of adults report feeling lonely.

Tell that statistic to many busy multitasking adults and they might say they'd do anything for some alone time, so context matters. Being alone is a normal part of life, but when this becomes feeling lonely, we know that this is an independent risk factor that negatively impacts our heart, brain and immune system.

Being lonely can be as harmful as a chronic disease. Thought to trigger a chemical stress response, lonliness can also activate our immune system as if we are managing a perceived threat. This makes sense, as humans were built to be social creatures and live and survive in groups and communities.

When loneliness becomes the normal state, stress and inflammation can impact how our brain cells function, in exactly the same way as chronic stress from other circumstances or disease can do this.

Loneliness is an independent risk factor for premature death of all causes, is strongly associated with cognitive decline and dementia and has been shown to be comparable to smoking 15 cigarettes a day. *Yikes.* The good news is that the opposite of loneliness is social connection, and this can be improved with even small gestures. A smile, a little bit of chit chat can be a mood lifter and alter the course of someone's day. Done enough, it can improve health, mood and means we are more likely to offer that same olive branch of communication to someone else.

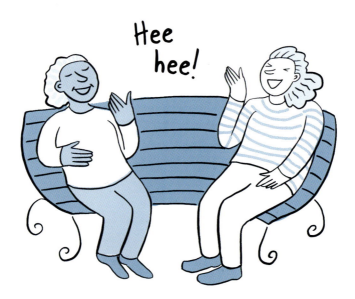

But what if you are surrounded by people, and still feel lonely?

When I was twenty-four, I had the opportunity to travel to New Zealand before I started GP training. Although solo travel felt terrifying, I knew that when I got there, I'd be fine, as several others from my university year group were already there.

But something totally different happened. Or rather, that was exactly what happened, but it didn't turn out the way I expected.

Despite being surrounded by friends I loved, having a flat to live in that was stumbling distance from local taverns and the beauty of New Zealand at every vantage point, I was absolutely miserable.

To counteract that feeling, I did more.

I made more plans for excursions, I said yes to everything (except bungee jumping). And yet the more I did, the worse I felt. To add to that I was panicking. Was this how I was going to feel forever? Was I depressed? I was on an extended holiday to the other side of the world, a once in a lifetime opportunity that I'd saved up for, so what the hell was wrong with me?

I was so unhappy in myself in New Zealand that I left early. I had booked a couple of days in Los Angeles to break the journey on the way home, assuming I'd be using the time to catch up on sleep after having so much fun. I began to centre myself before I got home and then straight into work. Still nervous of being alone, it took me by complete surprise that it was in the silence of properly being alone that I felt like I could breathe for the first time in weeks.

It's not just me.

Research has shown that loneliness was rated at similar levels both when people spend 75 percent of their time alone or the same amount of time with other people.

THE RELATIONSHIP WITH YOURSELF IS AT THE CORE OF EVERYTHING.

Accepting change

Changing relationships with the ones we love the most is the only certainty in life, yet we are still unprepared for it.

This can feel hard when we haven't experienced it before. Each child or parent is unique and with that comes individual challenges. Our brain likes to find the familiar. We see our parents age and our children grow up and it can be hard to remember that we are changing too. Our brain is fuelling this change as it ages but with that can come resistance. Thinking and managing the changes that are happening, both around us and within us is exhausting. Our brain knows that. So, it can be easier to stick with the familiar.

We wear the same clothing even though they don't look quite the same on our changing midlife frame.

We cook the same recipes our kids always loved without considering they might be open to something spicier or more textured than when they were five.

We see our partners and friends in the same way we did when we first knew them. Even if that was twenty years ago: we hark back to the person they were then rather than the anxious, stressed person that is front of us.

Change in relationships can take place gradually and quietly as children grow up and parents age. It can also come banging on your front door when there is a pivotal moment of loss.

How to make better friends with yourself

Talk to yourself!

Research shows that this is the opposite of crazy and has been shown to:

- Reduce anxiety

- Improve motivation

- Improve mood

- Help with planning and give you a bit more company

- Improve verbal working memory (for example, it helps you remember what you need before you leave for a trip or as you go through a store).

Knowing that this can feel hard and scary is important.

Our brain is problem solver, it wants to get to a solution asap but that isn't always possible. Sitting in the unknown is ok, we don't have to have the answer right now about how to deal with a boundary-challenging teen or a parent that isn't managing at home as well as they used to.

Resistance vs acceptance

Here are some familiar lies we tell ourselves on a mission of self-protection.

'He's fine.'   'No, I'm not annoyed with you.'
'Yes, that invitation sounds lovely, thank you so much we can't wait.'

Research has shown time and time again that acceptance, especially self-acceptance, is what makes the difference when it comes to feeling better in ourselves and being able to find the solutions we need.

If you're struggling with this, my recommendation is to sleep on it – sometimes you have to go to bed angry or worried. Sleeping can soothe our stress hormones, calm our thoughts and help us see any situation more clearly. Even if we don't dream up the perfect answer, whatever relationship quandary you are grappling with, it will feel better once the brain has rested and been through hours of sleep.

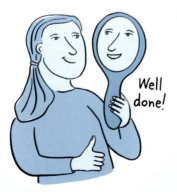

Well done!

Listen to what you are telling yourself

If it feels negative a lot of the time it's maybe a sign that these words need to be heard by someone else who can help you work through why this is the case. Being happier alone doesn't mean you don't like your friends or your partner, it just means you need time and space to hear yourself.

Post-sleep responses to those lies we tell ourselves:

'I'M WORRIED ABOUT MY DAD.'
'I LOVE YOU BUT YOUR INABILITY TO PLAN THE FAMILY CALENDAR WITH ME IS ANNOYING.'
'THANK YOU BUT WE CAN'T MAKE IT.'

This works both ways: Sometimes it's the acceptance part that is the problem.

Having a chronic illness where fatigue is at its core, primarily impacting my brain function and energy levels, I have had to learn this the hard way.

My default mechanism was always: 'Yes, sounds great, I'll do it.' Eventually though, I got to a point where my body and brain could not keep up. And given the nature of my health I know that situation can return at any time so balancing how I feel, physically and mentally in situations and with people has become a skill I've had to learn and keep relearning.

Relationships have a huge effect on our immune systems

The truth is that we are all just a big mish-mash of connections. Our brains are connected to our nervous system and our gut system AND all three are connected to our immune system. As a result, there's a field of research medicine called **psychoneuroimmunology** that is exploring just exactly how your mind, your brain, your nervous system and your immune system all interlink and have an impact on each other.

Data has shown that falling in love increases gene activity in antiviral defences. Conversely, when we feel insecure in close relationships, the data shows we exibit signs of weaker immune function.

Stressful relationships are more than just unpleasant to be in. They are harmful to our health: our mind, our brain AND our immune system all suffer.

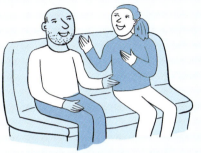

QUALITY OVER QUANTITY

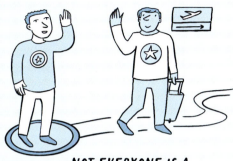

NOT EVERYONE IS A
BEST FRIEND FOREVER

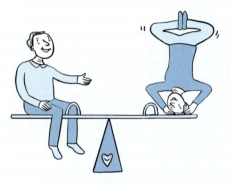

A HAPPY ROMANTIC PARTNERSHIP CAN
HELP US LIVE LONGER, HEALTHIER LIVES.
BUT THERE CAN STILL BE HARD TIMES

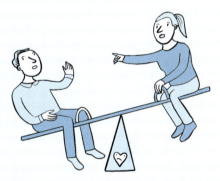

CHANGE IS INEVITABLE IN EVERY RELATIONSHIP

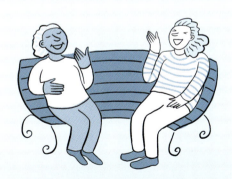

SOCIAL CONNECTION IS THE
OPPOSITE OF LONELINESS

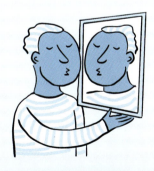

TAKE GOOD CARE OF
YOUR RELATIONSHIP WITH
YOURSELF!

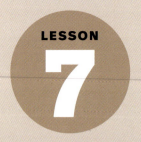

WALK, RUN, BOOGIE

OXYGEN + BLOOD FLOW + MOVEMENT = YOUR BRAIN'S SURVIVAL TRIANGLE

Movement and exercise are undeniably good for us. They help us live longer and be healthier, they improve our memory and thinking, reduce anxiety and depression, improve sleep and resilience and support a healthy immune system.

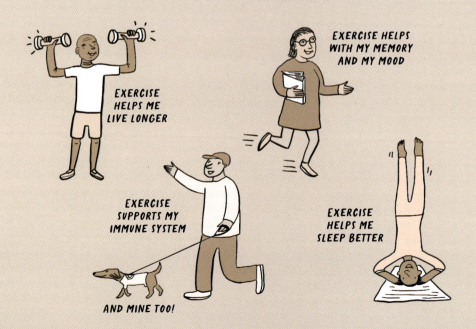

EXERCISE HELPS ME LIVE LONGER

EXERCISE HELPS WITH MY MEMORY AND MY MOOD

EXERCISE SUPPORTS MY IMMUNE SYSTEM

EXERCISE HELPS ME SLEEP BETTER

AND MINE TOO!

There is nothing that exercise cannot help. But why are over 50 per cent of women and 45 per cent of men not doing enough to achieve these benefits? To understand and go forward, we need to go back. Raise your hand if you enjoyed PE at school.

We form opinions about exercise and about our own exercise habits at a really young age. At school, within families and communities, the seeds of how we think about exercise and sport are sown when we don't even realise it.

This, of course, may change as we become teenagers and then enter adulthood – you only have to look at social media to see this. We have never had more choice of activities and platforms to monitor and challenge us. We can have instructors in our homes telling us literally what to do, and how to do it. But does this work?

Nothing will replace our personal motivation and the steps we take to transform this into action.

As life changes, so too does how we are able to exercise. Demanding children, menopause, life events, changing jobs, commuting, responsibilities can all make it harder for many of us to exercise than it was in, say, our twenties. Those few minutes we have to do something just don't feel like enough time to get over the mental hurdles. There's the voice of that teacher telling us we were rubbish at PE, there's the recollection of the feeling of being picked last for the team. And there are the hundred other things that we should be doing instead.

Make movement part of your everyday routine

We need to move more. That's a given. So the question 'Will I or won't I?' is moot. What you should really be asking yourself is '*How* can I move more?'

There are two ways to tackle this question. The first is to think about how you can introduce more movement into what you already do every day. At work, for example, you could use the bathroom two floors above rather than the one outside your office. You could set a reminder to get up every hour and have a walk instead of reaching for coffee and donuts. Your brain will love the creative challenge of finding little tricks to get you moving.

Second, there is Actual Exercise – we need to ask ourselves when we can move for twenty minutes today?

This could be in the form of a brisk walk, online yoga or a run around the block. Only you know the answer to what may work for you, but I do know that we all have twenty minutes that we can do this in.

Every. Single. Day.

The sitting problem

Inflammation begins in our muscles after only fifteen minutes of sitting. Not only that, but electrical activity in leg muscles reduces, fewer calories are burnt, insulin effectiveness decreases and the enzymes that help break down fat decrease by 90 per cent. Ninety per cent!

There is research aplenty on the specifics of exercise. If you get into regular exercise and want to up your game and learn more about what helps what and why, go for it and enjoy every moment. But if you are in the 50 per cent of adults who are not exercising, all the technical stuff can wait.

Get your twenty minutes in every day and take it from there.

Five and ten minutes are also good, but twenty is better.

Seven days of twenty minutes takes us very close to the one hundred-and-fifty minutes a week recommended guideline. And it's easier to fit in than thirty minutes. I don't know about you, but running for half an hour can feel like a lot when you haven't run since you were ten.

How do I know this? Because I have been there.

Never fast enough at school despite my best efforts, I got stuck on the stop of a scramble net on an assault course at fourteen and vowed that I'd never do anything like that again. And I didn't.

I joined gyms and never went.

I went to the odd exercise class in a community hall but was never able to keep up with the steps.

So, I gave up exercise FOREVER.

Then I was diagnosed with MS at thirty-three and, much to my annoyance, everything I read talked about the importance of exercise. Seven years post-diagnosis came Covid, and I walked, like everyone else, for around twenty minutes every day. And it wasn't that bad, after all.

So, I did other active things for twenty minutes a day and, before I knew it, as I approached forty-one, I was a Regular Exerciser.

Watching sport can be a (small) workout too

Regardless of which 50 per cent you are in, stats for watching sport prove we love watching it even if we've never picked up a ball, club or racquet. And watching sport can affect our brains.

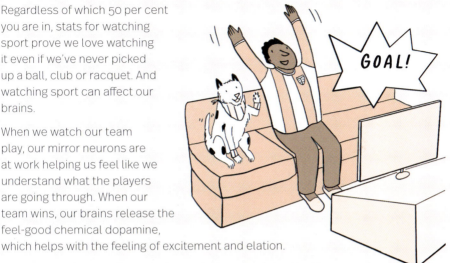

GOAL!

When we watch our team play, our mirror neurons are at work helping us feel like we understand what the players are going through. When our team wins, our brains release the feel-good chemical dopamine, which helps with the feeling of excitement and elation.

Conversely, when our favourite is on a losing streak, cortisol is released which can increase feelings of stress. Researchers have found that our brains can also reduce production of serotonin which can affect our mood and contribute to feelings of anger.

It's also not unusual for devout fans to feel anxious before a game. Sweaty palms, heart racing and some nausea are classic anxiety symptoms that are triggered in response to our brain's reaction to the build-up to a contest we care about. Our body can also produce adrenaline in response to these feelings which can increase heart rate and blood pressure.

Research done in Canada actually found that watching football can increase your heart rate to a level equivalent to a vigorous work out. At least as a spectator at home, if it all feels like it's getting too much, you can always change the channel!

What happens when we exercise?

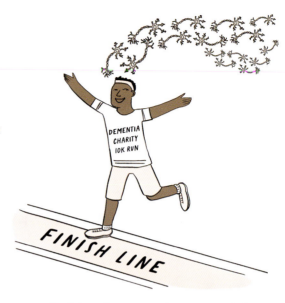

One session of exercise immediately increases the production of all those important life affirming neurotransmitters – dopamine, adrenaline and serotonin. Once you get past the 'this is too hard' stage, that's why you feel like you could write that novel, finally send that email you've been putting off and deal with that really annoying parent on the WhatsApp group head on. Because of these amazing impacts as a result of these hormones, there is a good chance you may actually get some of these things done, as concentration and focus remains at peak for at least two hours after exercise. And you are less likely to drop things after you exercise too, as that one session can improve your reaction time.

EXERCISE HELPS CREATE NEW BRAIN CELLS AND STRENGTHENS THE CONNECTIONS OF THE ONES YOU HAVE.

Exercising regularly is like a unique form of insurance policy as while it does hopefully protect your brain in the longer term, you don't have to wait until you are in your golden years to feel the benefits from it.

That brief improved attention span post-workout that helped you tackle 'that' task, can last beyond the post-workout haze when you exercise regularly: the brain area that helps improve your focus and concentration also improves then too.

An insurance policy

EXERCISING REGULARLY IS LIKE WEARING THE GUMSHIELDS WHEN IT COMES TO YOUR FUTURE BRAIN HEALTH.

Exercise encourages the growth of new brain cells that help our memory (improving and supporting our hippocampus) and strengthening the attention-focusing area of our brain (the prefrontal cortex). These are the areas that are most often impacted when it comes to age-related cognitive decline and Alzheimer's disease.

Please don't get me wrong: exercise *isn't* a wonder drug or a fix-all cure. It is a gumshield that you can use every day to protect your brain as you age. And you will feel the brain health benefits as you do it so it's not like an expensive insurance policy you are paying into for years thinking am I just wasting my time and money here.

Good news for the girls

In 2024, the Journal of American College of Cardiology found that women had the same longevity benefits from exercising 140 minutes per week vs 300 minutes for men. Why?

Women have higher density of capillaries per unit of muscle vs men, so they get more blood flow sooner with less exercise.

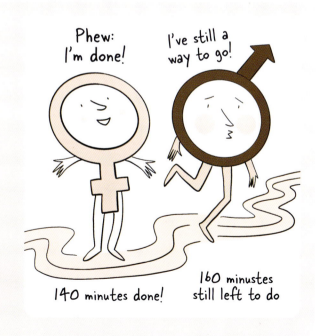

Phew: I'm done!

I've still a way to go!

140 minutes done!

160 minustes still left to do

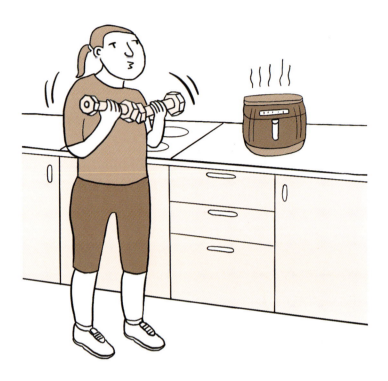

The motivation problem

We all know that exercise is good for us, so why do a lot of us (my hand is up) really struggle to enjoy it?

Appearances can be deceiving – just because we are dressed in active wear doesn't mean we all want to be active. Between our negative inner chatter about not being very good at it AND the actual physical effort needed to lace up and move, our energy saving brains are more than happy for us just to kick this can down the road and sit on our bums. You've also probably got a list of things you'd a) rather do, and b) have to do.

So how do we start to overcome this?

The running mice

Theodore G, a research scientist, wanted to get under the hood of these questions so as many great scientists do, he elicited the help of rodents.

He evaluated twenty-nine consecutive generations of mice to try to see if he could motivate each successive group to be more efficient and enthusiastic runners than the first. Given the equipment they needed, by generation 15 the mice were running 15km a day. By round 29, they had become the Usain Bolts of the mice world.

What had changed?

Their physicality improved as they ran more but the first breed of mice that became super runners couldn't claim they had runners' bodies. So how did they evolve? **The reward system** of the super runners' mice brains was the answer. They had a brain structure that showed an enlarged reward system so this was the carrot that kept them running. Once future generations had the physicality to match their runners' brains, boom, there was a gold medal waiting for each of them.

So, is it my grandparents' fault I never won anything at sports day?

Yes. And no.

Twin studies show 50 per cent heritability when it comes to physical activity. There is also a genetic link to how much you enjoy the exercise of 12 to 35 per cent.

We can influence this reward system, I promise.

When people become parents their reward system helps with an increase in grey matter within the brain in the first few months of their child's life. The more this area grows, the more positively they talk about their baby and their role as parents. These changes within the brain are very similar to what happens when people become regular exercisers. Our brain is built to help us exercise, it's our self-belief + genetics + distractions that keep us away from it.

That's why super runners talk about finding an activity they love,[1] because once they trigger that reward system, their brain takes over and helps drive them to maintain this habit.

THE WAY TO ENJOY EXERCISE IS TO DO IT.

---

[1] Or like. Or, at least, don't hate.

Tools to help you move

Find your own team

Any movement or exercise you do is great, but when you combine that with other people doing the same thing as you, all the benefits increase. We are built to live and grow together, and whether you are walking with a friend, in a virtual spin class or part of a dance group, making exercise a group effort increases every benefit exercise can bring.

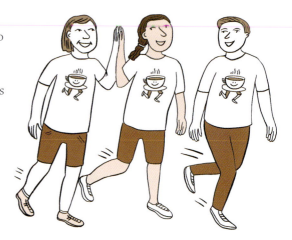

Find your beat Music is a legal performance-enhancing drug. Those are not my words but the findings from a review article from 2016 published in the *Annals of Sports Medicine and Research*. Whether it's the soundtrack to the movie *Rocky* or a classical playlist, music motivates us to move by reminding us of positive memories, mood supporting lyrics and a contagious melodic beat that makes us want to tap our toes and keep up.

Not convinced?

Every era has its own group dance track that captures us whether we want it to or not. What else could be the reason that phrases like 'Hokey Cokey', 'Macarena' and 'Cha Cha Slide' are making you want to clear the floor and move just by reading them. (Go on do it, no one is watching!)

Ignore yourself While listening to yourself about your health is one of the most important things I've discovered in all my years of being both doctor and patient, the one exception to this rule is when it comes to exercise and getting active. We are more likely to tell ourselves we can't do it about our physical ability than any other aspect of our lives. From a reformed exercise hater, know this – we *can* do it. Please don't abandon the benefits that exercise and movement can bring to you because of that memory from gym class. Or from being picked last for the team or coming last in the race. That said, if it actually hurts, don't ignore yourself. Take medical advice.

Don't overcomplicate it If you sit a lot for your job like most of us, stand up every hour. Two minutes of movement every hour has been shown to reduce your chance of dying by a third.

Mix it up Cardio, strength training and resistance-based work all have different benefits. But getting your heart rate up at least two to three times per week is where we see benefits in areas of the white matter of the brain that support memory and thinking abilities.

Health not weight Exercising solely to lose weight can be a losing battle. One reason for that is if you exercise regularly, you will build muscle and this weighs more than fat. There is a lot of research that shows exercise just isn't a good way to lose weight. However, as you know, when you exercise regularly you feel better, the reward cycle is activated, and this translates into other areas of your life to help you lose weight if indeed that is a goal for you.

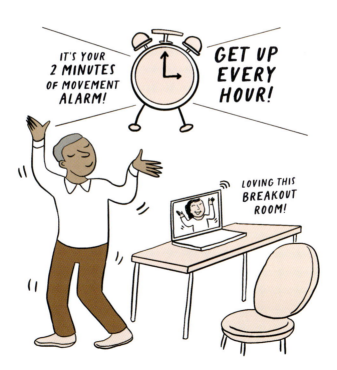

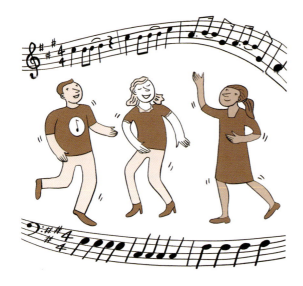

Moving your body, which is all that exercise really is, is about more than getting your heart rate up. It strengthens your muscles, builds brain cells, acts as that all important gumshield against age-related neurodegenerative disease.

It is an anti-depressant, an anxiety treatment and can make you immediately shimmy when you hear someone say, 'put a ring on it'.

IF THERE IS ONE TYPE OF EXERCISE THAT BRINGS IT ALL TOGETHER, IT'S DANCING.

Socially engaging, stress- and anxiety-reducing, endorphin-boosting dancing. Regardless of whether you cha-cha or kitchen shuffle, repetitive movement to music has been shown to improve working memory, improve pain thresholds and even reduce anger levels.

By thinking about steps and routines, we move out of set patterns of thinking and this not only improves energy, but it also reduces stress too.

The structural solution

Time slips through our fingers faster than sand. The best of intentions will go to dust and not build any sort of sandcastle without structural elements to your day in place to make them happen.

When – commit to a time in your day that you can do something active. You decide what you can manage in that time. Start today.

Write it down or buddy up – having something to help you stay accountable is helpful.

'But I . . .' – if you miss a day or a week accept that it happens. Start again. Today.

Reward yourself – your brain will do this for you, but it never hurts to have a little help in the beginning. Buy a new water bottle or create a cheesy playlist.

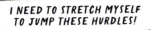

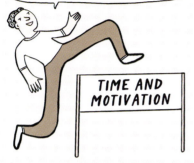

TIME AND MOTIVATION

ALL MOVEMENT COUNTS

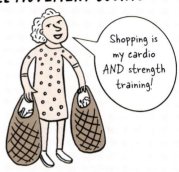

IT'S NEVER TOO LATE TO GET STARTED

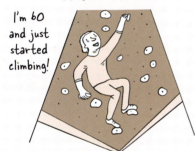

USE TECH TOOLS TO HELP YOU

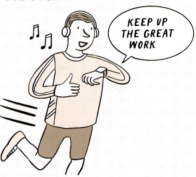

YOUR RELATIONSHIP WITH EXERCISE IS LIFELONG

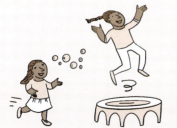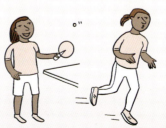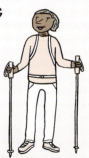

TAKE A TRIAL SEPARATION (IF YOU NEED TO), BUT DO START AGAIN

TICK, TOCK, BOOM

HORMONES — NOT JUST AT WORK BELOW YOUR WAIST

I'm going to take you back in time to school science and remind you of those pesky things called hormones. Defined as chemical messengers, they only got to work on their target organ, or so we thought.

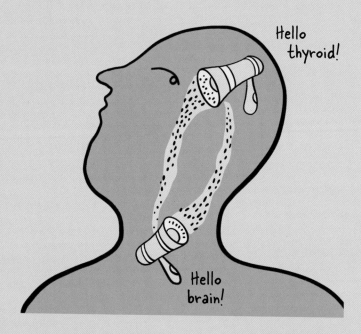

Hello thyroid!

Hello brain!

Thyroid hormones worked on the thyroid gland – that sits in the middle of your neck.

Oestrogen worked on ovaries and wombs to help women have babies and testosterone was a man thing that made you strong and helped women have those babies.

Yet, if it is that simple, why are we talking about hormones here, in a book that is about your head?

Hormones are, indeed, chemical messengers but what we have a better understanding of today is the fact that they exert their powers beyond their original target organ.

Thyroid hormones do indeed work on your thyroid gland but they also impact brain function.

Similarly, hormones that are made within your brain act on organs beyond their mothership.

Cortisol, the stress hormone we are all familiar with, is produced in the adrenal glands which sit above our kidneys, as a direct result of hormones originally made within an area of our brain.

The hormones/brain two-way street

In addition to that, processes that we know are linked to a decline in our health such as inflammation will also impact hormones, so this is a complicated circuit that has your brain right at the centre of it.

For women this is even more complicated (bet you aren't too surprised on that one), in part because hormones are in our DNA and the X chromosome (of which women have two and men one) is much larger than the Y chromosome – about 900 genes larger, meaning women with their XX chromosome have many, many more genes that are implicated in hormone production and subsequent brain activity than men.

It's important to mention first that there is a lot we don't know about women's brains because science hasn't really looked into them very much when it comes to research. For a long time, it was thought that the brains of men and women were pretty much the same and all that was different were the organs 'down there'.

Then at the other end of the spectrum were the narratives that told us male and female brains were from different planets.

Although there are still some moments where we might question it, the male and female brains and minds are from the same planet, and research continues into how they differ when it comes to everything from how we argue, to the roles of sex hormones in brain health and disease.

What we know, as of 2024:

Women...

are twice as likely to develop Alzheimer's dementia as men

have an increased risk of autoimmune diseases compared to men

are more likely to be diagnosed with depression than men

Men...

are twice as likely to develop Parkinson's disease

are more likely to develop non-Alzheimer's dementia (vascular or Lewy Body dementia)

are at higher risk for diagnosis of ADHD

die by suicide almost four times more than women

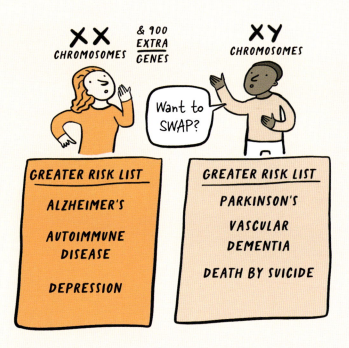

Reducing the causes for these changes to all being hormonal would be a gross oversimplification and instead we need to be having conversations that are going to help us understand more about potential solutions

Oestrogen and our brains

- Regulates glucose metabolism – the fuel your brain uses to function
- Regulates your mood
- Helps control body temperature
- Protects brain cells from ageing
- Supports your immune system

'Don't mind me, I'm just hormonal'

The fact is that women are *always* hormonal since our brains are constantly responding to a cycle of change that begins in early puberty and takes us all the way through our lives post-menopause. That is around sixty years of '*being hormonal*'.

Research published in 2017 shows that women's brains begin to slow down in functioning as we move from perimenopause into menopause, and beyond. Researchers studied how glucose, our brain's primary fuel, was metabolised within our brain and the results showed around a 20 per cent reduction in this process.

Why? The answer appears to lie in the role and function of oestrogen.

The monthly cycle

Now we understand more about oestrogen and its role in our brains, it is a bit easier to comprehend why it can impact our mood, energy and thinking on a cyclical basis.

Research is showing that the during follicular phase (days 1–14 of the menstrual cycle), women feel more energised, outgoing and have more energy, while during the luteal phase – post-ovulation – this can change as we get closer to the onset of the period and we become more irritable, withdrawn and less likely to want to socialise.

Stress, illness and difficulty sleeping can impact these stages, making the difference between the points in the month feel more noticeable and having more of an impact on day-to-day life.

Recognising that these changes in how we feel are indeed hormonal and cyclical can be helpful. Talking to our doctors and having a clear idea of what happens throughout the months can be helpful to determine how to improve how we feel.

The female brain is always changing

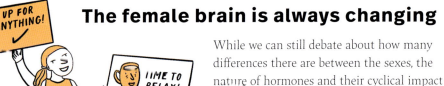

While we can still debate about how many differences there are between the sexes, the nature of hormones and their cyclical impact on our brain function is clearly different thanks to oestrogen and its partner in crime, progesterone.

Menopause

When oestrogen levels drop as women move through their forties and fifties, symptoms occur to let you know that your hormonal tides are turning.

While the changes in periods are the textbook ones that GPs were taught to ask about, me included, we know now that it's all the other stuff that causes more problems. Hot flushes, insomnia, dry skin, vaginal dryness, lack of libido, irritability and mood changes, memory lapses, brain fog, slower thinking, lack of motivation, weight gain AND changes to your bathroom habits.

I could go on – snoring, heartburn, burping . . . but I'd run out of pages. The common denominator in all these symptoms is oestrogen. And where does oestrogen have the most impact? In the brain. So, it's your brain that causes those hot flushes.

Testosterone

Seen as a male sex hormone, testosterone has important roles for both men and women.

While men do go through hormonal changes, the andropause or male menopause, where their hormone function also alters, is not thought to have the same impact on male brains as the equivalent has in females. These hormone levels decline much more gradually (which is why Robert de Niro can still become a new dad in his eighties) and the decline that does occur is comparatively symptom free.

Men's oestrogen levels (yes, men *do* have oestrogen too) will decline as well, but also at lesser levels, and testosterone production will compensate for this in their brain function, meaning men do not experience the symptoms women that have during menopause.

How to support your brain during menopause

1 Talk to your doctor about HRT – we know that replacing the declining hormones is the most effective way to improve all these symptoms. You may choose not to take it or be unable to take it for other health reasons but talk to your doctor and understand what is available to you.

2 Prepare yourself – take a diary of your symptoms and how you feel. No doctor intentionally dismisses or ignores symptoms, but we know unfortunately this happens too often.

3 Care for your vulnerable brain – midlife brings challenges that are the exact opposite of what you need when your brain is not at its best. Knowing this and proactively supporting yourself during this time is one the most helpful things you can do. Sleeping, moving, managing your stress and eating the most nutrient-rich diet you can manage has never been more important.

4 It's a change not a death sentence – you made it through puberty, you've made it through years of monthly cycles. If you've been pregnant you know mum brain feels very real. Life looks different on the other side of these changes, yet, you've done it for years, and flourished. You can do it again.

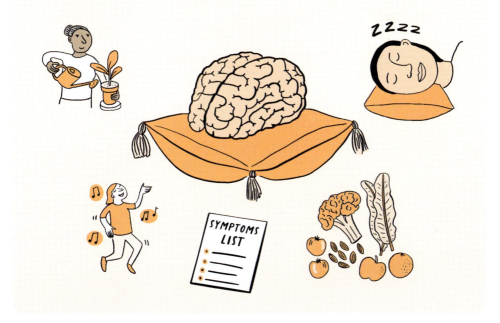

These sex hormones influence brain chemicals differently:

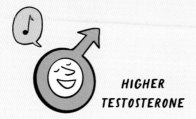

HIGHER TESTOSTERONE

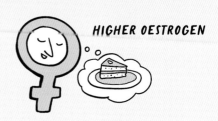

HIGHER OESTROGEN

Men (higher levels of testosterone) – produce more 'feel good' serotonin

Women (higher levels of oestrogen) – produce more 'reward motivated' dopamine

Sight

Men – have more M cells within the brain area that helps us see (visual cortex), which impact how eyes process movement

Women – have more P cells, which identify colour and shape

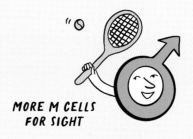

MORE M CELLS FOR SIGHT

MORE P CELLS FOR SIGHT

And if you ever thought the men in your life had 'selective hearing' there might be a reason for this

Women have over 10 per cent more brain cells in the area of our brain responsible for hearing. Which is why we are absolutely justified in telling our kids, we **can** hear everything.

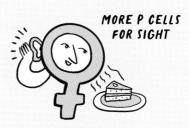

& OVER 10 PER CENT MORE BRAIN CELLS FOR HEARING

Your vulnerable brain

As hormonal changes occur over midlife, for both men and women, your brain becomes more vulnerable. We know that biological changes linked to Alzheimer's disease begin around this time. While the symptoms of Alzheimer's dementia may not reveal themselves until much later, helping people confuse these as part of 'normal ageing', all the evidence now shows us that this much feared condition is a disease of midlife.

Are hormonal changes a cause for this? Especially for women, given the protective role of oestrogen? Less oestrogen, less brain cell protection.

We don't fully know the answer to that yet and it's likely, as is the case in everything in medicine and health, not to be that clear cut.

However, the decline in oestrogen, and the symptoms this creates, can further increase the vulnerability of our brains to other conditions, as well as Alzheimer's.

For example, insomnia and hot flushes can impact our sleep which can, in turn, impact our mood, energy and food cravings.

Whether hormone replacement is an option for you or not, there are other ways we can provide extra TLC to our brains during this time of change.

Food The fuel we use is even more important now. Starting each day with a protein-filled breakfast along with increasing our fibre and healthy fat intake are at the cornerstone of this. Reducing caffeine can help with anxiety and all can reduce the blood sugar rollercoaster that can come from the hormonal, stressed, exhausted place we can find ourselves in, frequently without even realising it.

Sleep The dark forces may be at work to flip-flop our sleep patterns, but we can still improve this. Exposure to daylight before mid-day, no caffeine after 1 p.m. and trying to avoid that pre-bed nightcap are essential to improving your routine. Seek help if these are not working. Don't suffer in silence.

Stress management If you haven't already noticed, there is a lot to make your blood boil by the time you already in the throes of oestrogen decline. Developing a meditative practice is important to help you manage your stress levels. It doesn't have to be sitting cross-legged chanting (although that does work); many other repetitive simple tasks can provide a similar type of stress relief, including colouring, gardening or even ironing.

Nutritional supplements As a GP, I was always under the impression that there was no need to supplement your diet unless you had a clear deficiency. As a patient who experienced frustrating fatigue, my view on this changed once I began researching if and how supplements can be helpful.

Even with the best of intentions, most of us do not eat an optimal diet every day (if we've even figured out what that actually is). Once we do sit down to eat there are still unknowns when it comes to what is on our plate including how well our gut is absorbing these nutrients and the nutrient content of the food we have in front of us.

In 1950, a single orange would have provided our daily dose of vitamin A. Today, due to changes in soil quality and farming processes, we'd need to eat 21 oranges to get that same intake according to data published in the US in 2007.

Iron content in meat has reduced by up to 50 per cent, and essential minerals such as calcium and magnesium are down in everyday vegetables such as carrots and broccoli by 75 per cent. Research published in 2020, looking at dietary vitamin intake across countries including the UK, US and Germany found that intakes of multiple vitamins were below recommendation in significant numbers of the population across data from all countries. Up to 75 per cent of adults were deficient in some nutrients including vitamin D.

Do your research and talk to your doctor and qualified nutritional experts if this is something you are wondering about for you.

If you do invest in supplements, look at the ingredients list first, and if there are ingredients that are not the nutrients you want to be taking and you don't know what they are, think again. Fillers and additives are commonplace in the supplement industry and these ingredients at best offer you no benefits and can even sometimes give you side effects. And please ignore the 'menopause approved' label that is appearing on everything from tea to chocolate.

The ingredients are what matters, not what a marketing label says.

Putting the keys in the fridge again – is that normal?

Research points to the idea that brains shrink about 5 per cent per decade from the age of 40.

As we hit our fifties, the cortex, the outer covering of your brain, is becoming thinner, the protective myelin sheath coating the nerves is also thinner and this can impact the speed at which signals are fired and recovered between brain cells.

Mid-life Shopping List:

PROTEIN

GREEK YOGHURT · TOFU

FIBRE

BEANS · OATS

NATURE'S OESTROGEN

APRICOTS · CHICKPEAS · SESAME SEEDS · GREEN BEANS

HEALTHY FATS

SEEDS · MIXED NUTS · OLIVE OIL

DARK CHOCOLATE

70%

VITAMIN D

VITAMIN 'D'

What this means in real life is that on-demand recall of names and numbers, rapid task switching and processing speed can begin to decrease, as well as a slight decline in episodic memory (which is perhaps the reason you can't quite recall who said what in the meeting last week).

Yet, the good news is that wisdom, regulation and how we process the world around us continues to improve, or at least stay stable, with ageing.

Into our sixties, the ability to access our lifetime's worth of wisdom can be noticeably slower.

If these memory slip-ups and challenges begin to consistently interfere with everyday life it is time to be concerned and take action.

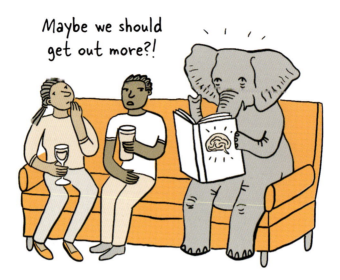

The elephant in the room

Being diagnosed with Alzheimer's is at the top of the list for health-related fears for adults over the age of fifty. Rather than living in fear, we can empower ourselves to care for our brains to reduce our risk of developing this condition. Think it's all in your genes? The reality is that very few cases of dementia are genetic in origin and even if you have genes that make your more likely to develop AD, your lifestyle can still pay a vital part in reducing that risk.

Forty per cent of all diagnoses of Alzheimer's dementia have been attributed to lifestyle associated risk factors. These include smoking, movement, high blood pressure, obesity, diabetes, low social contact, excess alcohol, hearing impairment and low educational attainment.

Treatments for Alzheimer's disease are on the horizon and closer than ever, but these are not yet curative.

It's never too early or late

Caring for your brain is the most powerful tool you have in keeping your brain healthy, even in the face of unknown brain-health threats such as Alzheimer's disease. As hormonal changes become permanent as we move through midlife, this is a really important time to start prioritising your brain health.

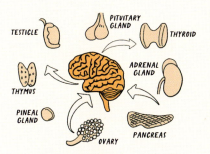

OUR HORMONES HAVE AN IMPACT ON OUR BRAIN HEALTH AND VICE VERSA

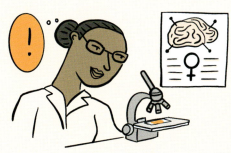

THERE'S A LOT MORE TO LEARN ABOUT FEMALE HORMONES AND BRAIN HEALTH

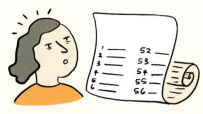

AS OESTROGEN DECLINES DURING MENOPAUSE OUR MOOD, MEMORY, SLEEP AND ANXIETY LEVELS MAY BE AFFECTED

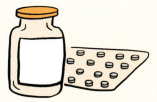

HRT CAN HELP WITH SYMPTOMS; TALK TO YOUR GP

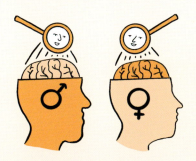

PREVALENCE OF ALZHEIMERS IN MEN AND WOMEN'S BRAINS AND THE ROLE OF HORMONES IS A FOCUS OF CURRENT RESEARCH

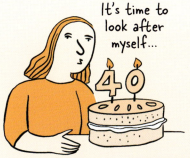

It's time to look after myself...

PRIORITISE BRAIN CARE AT MIDLIFE AND BEYOND TO HELP HOW YOU FEEL AND LOWER YOUR RISK OF ALZHEIMER'S

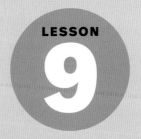
LAUGH, GIGGLE, PLAY

The opposite of play isn't work, it's death.
(Brain cell death that is.)
What do Tina Fey, *Friends*, *Fawlty Towers* and
a baby biting a finger all have in common? In
recent years they have all been voted the funniest
in their category. Why is that important?

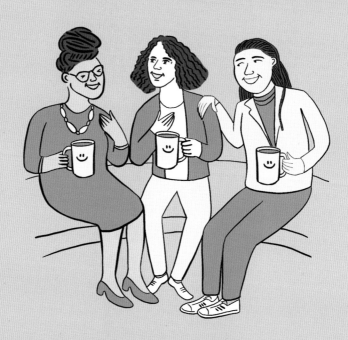

Turns out finding humour and expressing laughter are powerful tools for our brain and overall health. It's not all about entertainment.

What is laughter?

Laughing is an innate ability we are born with. Children who are deaf and blind still laugh. My brother has severe learning disabilities and cannot speak, however when he laughs, which thankfully he does often, you cannot help but smile. It is the sound of pure joy.

Laughing isn't really about how good the joke is. It is a social emotion influenced by community and relationships. To find something funny, we need to see something in the outside world and process it through our brain's internal workings, then represent it to our mind before we can initiate a smile, giggle or tear-inducing laughter. Thankfully, that process all happens in microseconds, or stand-up comedians would be performing for hours. Laughter experts (yes, that is a real job) know that our emotional state influences what, and if, we can find the humour in the joke.

WHEN WE LAUGH, GOOD THINGS HAPPEN WITHIN OUR BRAINS.

Endorphins are released and this triggers mood-lifting serotonin. Cortisol is reduced, which encourages perspective, improves problem-solving and stimulates creative thinking. Laughing improves our immune system and, if it's really funny, gives us our tummies and upper body a physical work out. Laughing helps reduce blood flow and blood pressure.

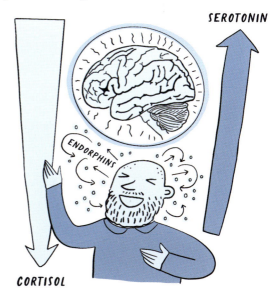

MRI scanners have shown that exposure to laughter in animal testing triggered a response in an area of the brain responsible for preparing facial muscles for expression. In this case, a smile.

Researchers concluded that this is part of why we smile in group situations when we see something positive happening.

Humour as a therapeutic tool

When it comes to our brains, seeing something as funny is a two-way street. If we are in a good mood, it is easier to find something funny than if we are feeling very negative. However, sometimes when we are at our lowest and we least expect it, something that we shouldn't find funny, is. And this release of laughter helps us feel better, even if is only temporarily.

Not finding humour in things that you normally would be a sign that your mental health is not at its best.

Patch Adams, the US doctor made famous in the Robin Williams movie of the same name, is more than just a screen hero. As a medic, comedian and activist, he has made it his life's work to help and heal others in a somewhat non-conventional way.

He has long considered clowns to have a similar role to doctors when it comes to their ability to reduce suffering. By recruiting clowns – aged 3–88, no screening process, anyone can apply – and bringing them to areas of deprivation, suffering and conflict, Adams uses humour to bring healing even in the most unthinkable circumstances.

Write your own laughter prescription

Having a laugh can provide instant therapy and relief. There might not always be a clown, or your favourite comic nearby so have a bank of things you find funny on standby for when you just really need a laugh.

YouTube clips, links to TV shows you love, photos that remind you of the time your husband walked into the lamp post just after you'd had an argument on holiday.

Injecting some silliness can also provide an antidote to fear and anxiety. That noise that you know is nothing but still creeps you out at night? Give it a name and imagine it as something totally different. That helps us disassociate the sound from being something to be scared of and changes the connection on our minds when we hear it the next time.

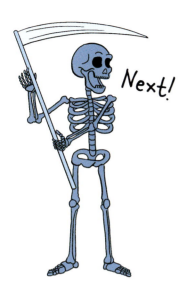

Next!

We use humour to cope with the unthinkable

Recently I attended a very traditional funeral. Everyone was in black; the service was religious and led by a priest.

As the pallbearers lowered the coffin into the ground, there was that horrible sense of finality that was clear by the audible silence.

Until three of the pallbearers lost their balance, fell into the grave and landed on the coffin.

The shrieks of horror and panic echoed through the crowd and those of us closest turned our heads away to avoid seeing what the aftermath of this may be. Thankfully they were young, fit men who pulled themselves out in seconds, unhurt and dusted off the mud from their black suits.

It took almost an hour for this to translate from horrific to a quiet source of humour for some of the funeral goers. By teatime, we were talking of the saddest of losses and the humour of the grave fall in the same sentence.

This gallows humour is a way of coping in dark moments and a stress aid that has been used for centuries to help us come to terms with the unthinkable.

Known as the relief theory of humour, the concept is that these unthinkable moments can be funny as they shock us from what are considered acceptable norms.

What is Play?

Play is purposeless, voluntary and builds a sense of anticipation.

Play creates freedom from time, a reduced awareness of oneself and a desire to continue.

It is impossible to think of what play is without thinking of how it makes you feel. Joyful, light, free, happy.

Play is something that we are naturally drawn to. There is a really good reason for that. You see, we need to play to survive.

Nobel Laureate and neural scientist Gerald M. Edelman created a theory on how new information is integrated into our brain cells. Essentially, new things are coded into our brain cell function in 'maps', which help our neurons link together. This is the reason we recognise groups of different types of objects and know what they are. This is why we know a road is a road and not a sea.

Once we have these basics in place we also start to layer in emotion and memory, which adds textured layers to something that was once a simple structure. (That was the road we used to walk along to get to school, remember that day it was snowing and we had a snowball fight? and so on.)

The mapping of these recognition pathways and how we interpret them throughout our lives, change. They are not fixed. The more experiences we have, and the more we experience emotion and create memories in these different settings, the better we are preparing ourselves for possible eventualities.

Real or imagined? Both count

The make-believe games and relationships with imaginary friends that we enjoy as children can form foundations for our ability as adults to daydream about our future or think about how we respond in conversations.

A strong theory of why play is important throughout our lives is that all these purpose-free joy-filled moments that we enjoy during this time positively impact these brain cells connections and wider networks.

If you are still on the fence about why play matters, remember this:

Core survival functions of life – breathing, consciousness and the drive to sleep – all originate in our brain stem. Guess what? Play researchers (yes, that is a real job, too) have worked out that play originates from there, too.

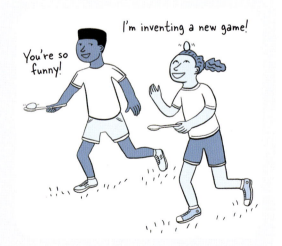

One theory of why play is important at every age is that by creating these joy-filled moments, not in the pursuit of a specific goal or purpose, we are both having fun and fuelling brain cell connections.

When we play and imagine, we are creating versions of possible outcomes while essentially test-running what might happen without any consequences. This helps prepare us for when reality strikes.

Peak playtime is when we don't even realise we are doing it. Research from studying rats in the 1960s showed that it wasn't just putting rats in playful bright environments that benefitted their brain cell growth, it was giving them toys and other rats to play with that really created significant differences. Although the research focused on animals, this proved that play is an extremely important way to help brain-cell networks create themselves.

While vast brain-cell growth and connection occurs during childhood, our ability to impact our brain-cell networks remains an active opportunity throughout our whole lives. When we look at research into patients with Alzheimer's disease, we see that those who remain engaged and mentally active maintain a higher quality of life, and even have a reduced risk of being diagnosed with this condition.

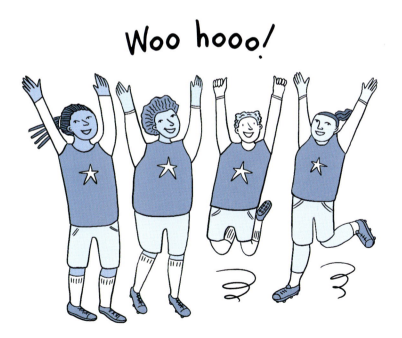

Science lesson over: let's play

One of the many benefits of social media is that there is now a very visible platform for people to talk about how, why and how fast they run/exercise/walk. We are obsessed with telling everyone with what we are doing and while that is good for the algorithms and engagement metrics, how good is it for us and our play brain?

REMEMBER HOW TO RUN LIKE PHOEBE

There is a key moment in *Friends* when we see Phoebe 'fun running' – with her arms and legs flailing and flapping, as opposed to moving in the conventional running manner. Embarrassed by this, Rachel decides to run alone until, one day, she decides to give fun running a go. Although she ends up backing into a horse, Rachel realises that running in the Phoebe way is actually a lot more fun.

For your exercise time to be considered play time, remember it has to be fun, have a sense of purposelessness and bring a reduced awareness of oneself.

If you are posting your latest physical achievement on social channels, check in with yourself – are you playing or posting about playing? They are different things.

How to Play

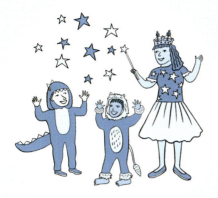

Spend time with kids and pets – their enthusiasm and ability to make everything silly, funny and a game is good for us grumpy adults, too.

Think back to your childhood and think about what activities brought you that sense of childlike joy. Ask yourself why you don't do any of those things now. Fair enough, having make believe tea parties with dolls or running through a sprinkler dressed in a bin bag (two of my particular favourites) may have practical limitations but the essence of those activities can be rediscovered as an adult play activity.

Throw a tea party for your real-life friends, have a theme, don't fuss about the food, just focus on the fun.

Allow yourself to be a beginner again. Playing a musical instrument, trying a new sport or something you haven't done since you were a kid are great ways to play. Relax, have fun. No one really cares if you're any good.

Not every aspect of a playful activity will be fun – but it could still be worth doing.

Cooking a new recipe might be a playful activity to try that needs preparation and planning. There is also no guaranteed success at the end. But approaching it with a playful attitude will make it fun regardless of whether there is a soggy bottom or not.

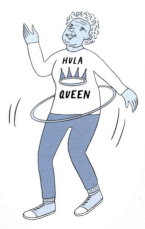

If all of this makes you cringe and want to pull a blanket over your head, the sure-fire way to bring play into your brain is to **get active**. Once we are freer in our bodies, this translates to our minds.

And remember, no one is watching you.

The only eyes on you are your own. So relax and just have fun.

Does watching a movie or reality TV count as play?

I don't think many of us would think of watching the news as fun. Even conflict-laden dramas or nightmare-inducing psychological dramas may have questionable benefits in the play department. But there is one type of TV that unquestionably brings the joy and it shouldn't be a surprise if you read the start of this chapter: comedy.

Don't Play to win.

Whether it is performing on stage or competing in a sports competition, the play brain benefit comes from the way that the activity makes you feel. If you ruminate for ages over losing a game or messing up your lines, this changes how your brain interprets these activities.

As the director Baz Luhrmann says: 'In the end it's called A Play because (we) play.'

When I overheard a teacher talking openly to a group of parents about which of the eight-year-olds in the class were 'the sporty ones', I wish I'd known about the work of sports coach and psychologist Gary Avischious. He works to counteract the 'A team' mentality that can sound the death knell for too many kids and their interest in and enjoyment of sport. When coaches and parents focus solely on winning, the only person that loses is the child. Avischious says, 'I brought the concept of play sciences into youth sports and saw how that changed kids' performance.'

Why does that work?

When the kids are fully engaged, they have fun and are more likely to learn the skills of the game. They also learn to laugh at themselves and not take it all so seriously.

If you think playing games instead of using drills to learn techniques is 'too soft', the proof is in the pudding: Gary's teams had a thirteen-year winning streak.

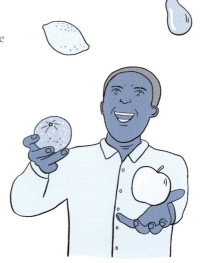

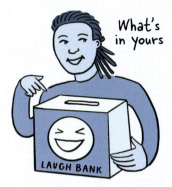

CREATE YOUR OWN LAUGH BANK
FOR WHEN YOU NEED A GIGGLE

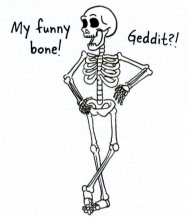

HUMOUR IS A POWERFUL TOOL WE USE
TO CONNECT AND SHARE EXPERIENCES

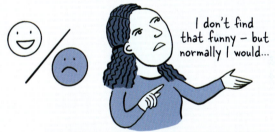

A CHANGE IN THE WAY YOU INTERPRET HUMOUR
MAY REFLECT YOUR CURRENT EMOTIONAL STATE

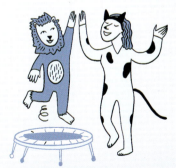

PLAYTIME ISN'T JUST FOR KIDS!

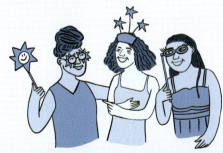

PLAY LIKE NO-ONE'S WATCHING

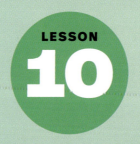
FEEL, CRY, FROWN

LET'S TALK ABOUT YOUR FEELINGS

This might be the scariest thing you face today.
Feelings run parallel to every moment of our waking lives.
They change from moment to moment and depend on
so many different factors. From our energy level, to how
hungry we are, to how we feel about ourselves.

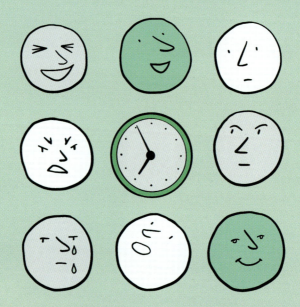

Thankfully, clever people have been studying these invisible things that determine so much of our lives for centuries and have some pretty clear ideas about why emotions and feelings matter so much.

Charles Darwin established that emotions were signals of important information that could influence behaviour to support our survival. Fear being the key here.

But then researchers realised there was a lot more to these than just keeping us from danger and began to look at thinking and behaviours and how our feelings influence these.

The phrase 'emotional intelligence' encompasses this and more – the idea that how we process our own emotions and those of others can steer our intelligence and how 'successful' we are in life.

Avoidance

How we feel matters to every aspect of our lives. So why do we do and say so much to avoid how we feel?

The fiftieth time you've checked your phone by 10 a.m.

Eating your way through the whole bag of crisps rather than 'just a couple'.

That surge of fury that surfs through you when someone says something to annoy you and you smile back, laugh and say something like 'yes that is SO true' when what you are thinking is a lot less PG-rated.

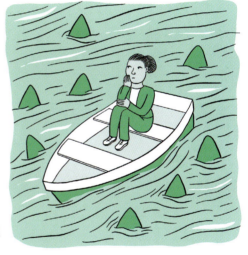

Emotions and feelings are scary. Especially the negative ones. Because they can make us vulnerable, fearful and as if we are stranded in a rowboat without paddles. We haven't been taught to deal with them. We aren't born knowing how we feel or what to do when these emotions take hold. Most of the time we don't even know what they are. We watch and learn and digest those around us and what they say or do. We take what we've seen and roll on with our own experiences, merge them with those we spend our time with and ta dah, we have a mish-mash of how we deal with feelings.

Once we become more aware of what is going on, and less fearful of these feelings, these emotions can actually become the paddles that can help us row to where we need to go.

Getting to know our feelings

Pixar's *Inside Out* won an Oscar for best animated feature, and *Inside Out 2* grossed one billion dollars in the first month of opening. We want to learn about our emotions, but ideally in a cute, funny animated way.

Within our brains, feelings impact the release and suppression of different neurochemicals. At the core of this is the HPA (hypothalamic-pituitary axis) which connects our brain to our hormonal system. Stress influences these pathways and brings about a nice circle of stress, hormones, emotions, mood. Where is the starting point to this circle? Hard to say, but by regulating our emotions and feelings, we can impact our stress response, which therefore can impact our mood, and yes, physical health.

Short bouts of stress strengthen these networks and improve emotional resilience.

Emotional resilience is a hot topic, especially when it comes to children and mental health. But it's important for adults too, and the truth is, many of us haven't really learnt how to compute our own feelings and how these translate into thoughts and behaviours. Essentially resilience is how we bounce back from difficult times. What we know from emotion researchers is that: a) acknowledging how we feel in the hard moments helps us grow through them, and b) the stress we feel during these times is a positive part in this process.

Why?

We think that by acknowledging the difficulty we are feeling and accepting the stress this brings, knowing it will be temporary, this can reshape our thought patterns to realise that we will be ok. Once we realise we are *actually* ok, this new wiring embeds itself into our brains so that the next time we find ourselves in free fall our brain remembers this.

How emotions influence us:

- Decision making
- Relationships
- Health

- Performance and what we do
- They shape what we focus on, learn and remember

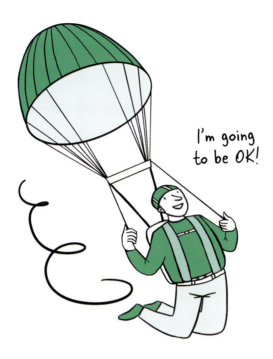

'HANG ON, WE'VE BEEN HERE BEFORE, USE THIS PARACHUTE AND WHILE THE FALL MIGHT STILL BE SCARY, I PROMISE YOU ARE GOING TO LAND SAFELY.'

If we never jump, or acknowledge that this process is scary and feels horrible, our brains never get to acclimatise to this type of stress and will only react to the feeling of falling.

The trick here is that we have to understand this and remind ourselves regularly for our brains to 'get it'. Our brains process our reactions and experiences in seconds to keep us safe. As a result, negative thoughts and emotions can quickly escalate, especially if adrenaline and cortisol are flying around. Which isn't always all that helpful (unless you have actually fallen off something).

We have to start with the small stuff. Let's talk about being late.

Disclaimer: my university yearbook named me: 'Just give me five minutes' Clara.

As I 'grew up' the biggest problem I faced when I ran late was how I spoke to myself as it happened and the subsequent fallout.

'YOU ARE GOING TO BE LATE, WHY DIDN'T YOU LEAVE EARLIER? YOU KNOW THE TRAFFIC IS BAD AT THIS TIME, YOU ARE GOING TO MISS IT, THEY WILL THINK YOU DON'T CARE, YOU WON'T GET THE CHANCE TO MEET THEM AGAIN, WHAT HAVE YOU DONE? WHY DIDN'T YOU LEAVE EARLIER?'

Meanwhile I was still trying to get there on time so I was making riskier decisions about driving or walking which could cause me physical harm.

By the time I was there apologising for being late, I was disappointed in myself and embarrassed which impacted the meeting time I had left. But it's too late at this stage as I was deeply entrenched in negative thought patterns about the situation and myself. When I eventually had a panic attack on a bus, I knew I had to change something.

I started with this mantra:

'NOTHING REALLY BAD WILL HAPPEN IF YOU ARE LATE TODAY.'

No one will die, given I'm not in primary school no one will shout at me and the absolute worst-case scenario is I miss it. Not ideal but fixable.

I reminded myself of this whenever I felt the flutter of my heart rate as I looked at the clock as I sat in traffic going to work, or school pick up. And most importantly, when I heard anyone I was with saying 'you are going to be late.' (Fyi that is NEVER helpful.)

Guess what? Now four times out of five, I'm on time.

Being aware of how we are interpreting what is happening within us means we can keep our brains' safety catch cycle for when we really need it.

Feeling more negative/anxious/depressed is associated with unhealthy behaviours that reinforce those negative thinking patterns. We can only focus on what we can do, which serves us better than ruminating over potential outcomes.

Does regulating emotion mean ignoring it?

No – quite the opposite. Most of us could get PhDs in ignoring our emotions. We can only regulate our emotions when we are aware of them.

If you aren't feeling great, good, awesome is that bad? Is something wrong with you?

No. We aren't designed to feel happy all of the time. Diagnosis – human living a normal life.

Emotions are barometers for what is going on within, yet we often do our best to dismiss or ignore them. If your foot was sore, would you keep running? If you feel nervous or angry, you owe it to yourself to stop and ask why.

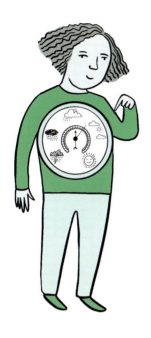

Your feelings matter, they help you identify what is going on within and that can help you make better decisions and care for yourself better.

When someone you love is crying it can be very difficult thing to watch. What do you do? Other people's tears can make us feel helpless and fearful. We like to fix and do things. Sitting in the sadness is not easy. But when we do, both for them and for ourselves, we can learn to become more compassionate and help ourselves face our own difficult emotions.

Being curious about our emotions makes us more likely to make decisions that are better for those emotions in the long run. When we ignore or suppress feelings, we are less likely to make the changes that benefit us, or even believe that we can make better decisions.

One word, different meanings

'I'M BORED.'

If you've been a child or had a child, you've heard this before. (Often the best answer is 'go and do something else then'?)

Boredom can mean you want to do something else – spark creativity – or it can mean you are exhausted and feeling overburdened, signifying it's time to take a break.

We have stock phrases.

Tiredness can actually mean sad. Or burnt out. Or angry. Psychologists call this 'clumping'.

One of the best examples of this is anger – lots of different things contribute to anger and not all of them are emotional. Having low blood sugar and being tired are two key physical experiences that are much more likely to make us feel or appear angry, especially to those who know us best.

Angry can also be a more socially acceptable interpretation of anxiety or frustration.

Some emotions roll off the tongue easily. But in your own mind, it can be useful to take an extra minute or two to think about if there is anything else physical or practical that you can do to change those emotions.

Physical things that can impact how we feel

Hydration – the brain feels the impact of dehydration before the rest of our bodies and it can't sound an alarm that says 'I'm thirsty'. Instead we can feel more irritable, or experience slower thinking and difficulty focusing.

Fuel gauge – many aspects of modern-day life require complex thought patterns and decision-making. These executive functions of our brain can be the first to be impacted when our blood sugar levels change, and this can impact our thoughts and emotions.

Pain – have you ever had a toothache and felt in the best mood of your life? Thought not.

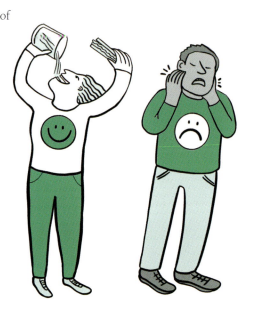

Physical pain hijacks everything rational thought – we think it will never end. Such is the intensity of the discomfort, it is impossible to think of anything else and we think it will always be like this. For those living with chronic pain, this can be extremely challenging.

The brain is wired to think unpleasant feelings are permanent, so what you can do to counteract that is narrow in on that feeling and remember we cycle through lots of emotions in a day. Even when we are in severe physical pain, we will experience a cycle of emotions along with the discomfort.

Self-regulation

Kids often use a blanket or cuddly toy to help them feel comforted and to enable them to regulate when they feel sad or worried.

Adults can do that too (although maybe bringing a cuddly toy into work with you might start to raise eyebrows) – a favourite mug, sweater or candle scent can help us feel safe and secure.

Bringing awareness to how we feel is the goal; to do that when our emotions feel like they are overpowering us takes practice.

We can use our own tools, as opposed to physical things to help regulate:

Say what you see – this immediately switches your focus from your feelings to the outside world so when you do return to your what's going on for your, the intensity has dialled down.

Go for a walk – movement and fresh air can also bring perspective.

Do something for someone else.

If in doubt, hum. You cannot ruminate on feelings or cry and hum at the same time.

When we can self-regulate, we can think more clearly and feel happier overall.

Children learn what they see. When you start regulating your emotions better, you are not only helping your mental health and brain health, but you are also helping that of your children too.

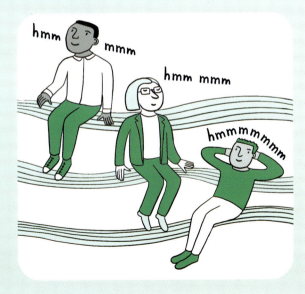

Strategies to manage difficult feelings:

Breathe slowly When it all goes wrong, our brain reacts to big feelings by firing up a fight, flight or freeze response. We breathe faster, our heart rate picks up and those stress hormones begin leaking everywhere. Remember this is all in an effort to keep us alive. But we can recognise this and slow the whole process down by taking some slow deep breaths. This calms the emergency warning system that has been activated and gives us time to pause before working out what to do next.

Plan ahead Family gatherings are the best example of when this can stop a boom or bust situation. You know what I mean. When you know something is a source of stress for you, plan how you can manage this the best way possible. Avoidance is at the far end of this spectrum, but a more realistic option might be adjusting a seating chart, ensuring if you are tired and stressed you keep contact to a minimum and know that you can always change your plans to do what is best for you and your health.

Change the channel You are being reprimanded unfairly at work and tied up in knots inside. You can stand up there and stare at your colleague who you know is trying to put you down in front of the boss or you can choose to focus on something else. Stand there and think of your shopping list for the weekend. The three songs that were on the car radio enroute to work. By shifting gears, we remove the emotion and dilute the feelings from those stress responses. This means when we move back out of neutral into second gear, we can show them our best selves.

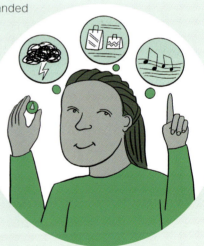

Clean the lens In my experience this can take a good night's sleep to be achievable. But it works. It isn't the same as dismissing the feeling, it is exactly as it sounds, cleaning the lens on how you are viewing a situation and reframing something into a different image. It almost certainly begins with: 'OK so what they said felt unfair and hurtful, but what can I learn / take / improve on / from this?'

Sharing is caring – or is it?

You know *that* person. They can't wait to tell you how amazing their life is, about their new kitchen, their partner's promotion, their kids' part in the school play. Perhaps you are that person. We can be great at sharing our own good news, and while that is important, we want to know we are safe to share the not-so-shiny things too in order to build real connections.

Working out when and with whom you can share those feelings with is important.

Not long after my son started nursery, keen to meet and make mum friends, I went for a coffee with a potential new friend and loved listening to her stories about how she met her husband, her mother's health scare and how she was unsure about her new boss at work. I saw this as true connection and eagerly shared my own current mindset, which at that time was full-on confusion on nearly everything due to my health and how this was impacting every aspect of my life.

When we parted, I felt I'd truly made a new friend and was so positive about sharing what I had. I felt lighter and more confident in myself. But when she wasn't free to meet again at various dates I gave her, I was left feeling upset and embarrassed. I'd shared too much of myself and I was angry at letting my guard down. People love sharing good stuff. But just because they share their bad stuff doesn't mean they want to hear yours.

I learnt a really hard lesson that day, and it held me back from being open when I met new people for a while. Knowing your emotions for yourself is the most important thing. When you feel ready to share them, choose wisely about who you allow in to see your deepest self.

The bee sting

You are rested, hydrated, stretched, exercised and you've breathed deeply.

Then something totally unexpected happens and you think you might just implode (or explode) on the spot.

Emotions and how they impact us are not linear. We are not Pixar characters. We are humans living complex and multi-layered lives. When the sting happens, sometimes the only thing you can do is flee. Walk away, hide in the toilet, cry in the car. It will pass, but for now, just do what you can to get through.

Workplace emotions

These are some of the hardest settings to navigate. I've heard patients talk about experiences in so many different work settings – from school canteens to national governments – that have similar difficult emotions in common.

Aren't we all scared to say what we feel to our boss? Even if they are super nice, should we really be doing that? What will they think?

Two things have been shown to matter here:

First, an emotionally aware culture led by at least one person with emotional awareness. (I know, I'm picturing places I've worked and struggling to come up with that person too.)

Second, feeling like you are heard – if a workplace can create an environment where their employees feel heard, even if the boss doesn't immediately act on what they are suggesting or can even fix the problems, feeling heard is more than half the battle.

Anxious? Join the club

When the animators at Pixar started to draw the Anxiety character for *Inside Out 2*, they struggled. Was Anxiety 'the bad guy'? Could Anxiety be both helpful *and* destructive? Or was she just a side character to fear?

I can understand why those creative geniuses found this hard.

First, we are talking about a spectrum of feelings and trying to define it in just one emotive word. There is feeling anxious about something specific at one end (which may not be pleasant but can be a reflex reaction to the unknown) to anxiety disorders at the other end (where anxiety is the dominant emotion in a person's life and influences all decisions and behaviours). Feeling anxious is a normal emotion that is essential to our survival and triggers the amygdala area of our brain to mount a fight or flight response. In a job interview setting, we can hopefully regulate this by focusing on doing the best we can as opposed to our sweaty palms and racing heart. Being chased down the street, feeling anxious focuses us on running the fastest we can to take flight from this actual threat.

But when anxious thoughts pop up in unpredictable situations, and mutate to thought loops that we can't switch off, this can evolve into a change in action or behaviour that has negative consequences for our overall life. We don't even apply for the job, or want to leave the house for fear of being chased.

When anxious thoughts are impacting your everyday life in a negative way preventing you from doing the things you want or need to do, talking to your doctor is the first step. From discussing therapies that gently question these thought loops and help you move to different patterns, to prescribed medication, help is there. Please take it. It's not 'just how you are'; anxiety disorders stifle potential and ruin lives. They can be managed and are extremely hard to tackle alone.

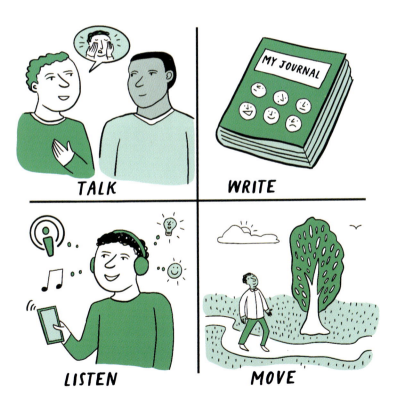

How to help dial down your everyday anxiety response:

Start by acknowledging how you feel – pretending negative emotions are not there only amplifies them

Slow deep conscious breaths – this slows down your fight or flight response and gives you some moments to think.

Try to identify what event or thoughts are driving this response.

Remind yourself that your current state is temporary. Even if the event or thoughts persist, how you feel and react to them can change.

What can you do now to stop these anxious thoughts in their tracks? Talk to a trusted friend, write down on a scrap of paper what just happened, focus on different sounds in your head – a piece of music, podcast or lace up and go for a walk.

Your Emotion Tool Box

Take a piece of paper and write these phrases down and then fill in the 'x':

What is the worst thing you think about yourself or a task/situation you are in?

I am x
This is x
I will never x
People think x

When you've done it, read it, then rip it up or burn it.

Now write these:

As a friend/child/parent – I am x
Three good things about me – x x x

Find a picture or a memento of you in this role that reminds you of these positive feelings.

Keep it safe.

One more thing: keep a folder on your phone of Pure Joy. Look at it whenever you need to.

The world we live in and our lives within it are unique to us all. We have the benefit of these tools to help us understand the what the why and what to do better but ultimately we must take what works for us and do the best we can.

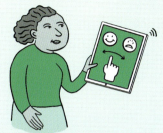

EMOTIONS PROVIDE IMPORTANT INFO, THEY ARE OFTEN FLEETING

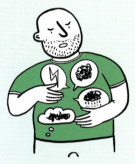

WE ARE HARDWIRED TO HOLD ONTO NEGATIVE EMOTIONS

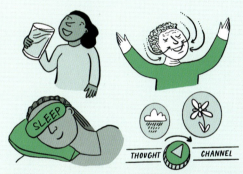

BUILD A STABLE FOUNDATION WITH GOOD HABITS IN ORDER TO INTERPRET EMOTIONS

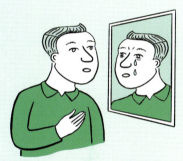

FACING HOW WE FEEL IS HARD

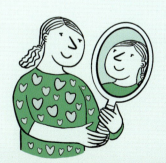

ACKNOWLEDGING OUR EMOTIONS CAN HELP US UNDERSTAND OURSELVES

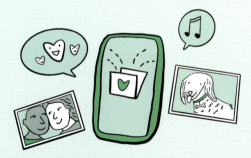

MAKE A FOLDER OF THINGS YOU LOVE ON YOUR PHONE

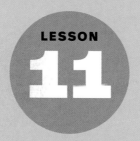

SAD, BAD, SURVIVAL

SOMETIMES WE JUST NEED TO DO WHAT WE CAN

The hardest thing about life is that when something really, really bad happens, everything else around us goes on.

The sun rises and sets.

The laundry basket continues to fill up.

And we still need to get stuff done.

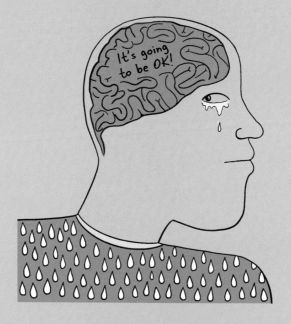

This is where our brain comes into its own. Remember its sole function is to keep us alive and keep us safe. So, although we may be feeling like things cannot get any worse, remember that our amazing brain will do its job expertly. It has been waiting for this moment.

We will be changed forever, but we will keep going and be OK.

Our brain will make us sleepy.

Remind us to eat or at least drink.

And if we eat or drink too much rubbish, that headache and nausea that appears will soon make us feel so much worse than we did in the beginning that we will put our poison down.

Those circadian rhythms that we talked about earlier in the book will keep everything ticking over in neutral until we are ready to move ourself back into first.

Numbing

Feeling sad is tiring and difficult and we will naturally do anything we can to numb these horrible feelings. While I do encourage you to feel your feelings, please remember that transient numbing is normal. It's totally OK to indulge yourself, but know that this is just a temporary fix and watch out for overspending, overeating or too much drinking because these are prolonged ways of coping that are just not good for us.

Our brain can only know how we feel, and that the dopamine rush that we get that feels SO much better than the swirl of sadness that was there before. But our brain doesn't really know if that rush is coming from a positive self-soothing behaviour such as having a nap, or a massive online spend that we can't afford.

Be alert.

Know how you are managing yourself and why, and watch for it in others when they are going through something tough.

DON'T UNDERPLAY THE BAD STUFF.

Sad

We think of grief as arising from the death of a loved one but, actually, we can grieve lots of different things, different endings and losses, and the impact on our brain is the same. It's still loss and represents a huge change from what we were expecting. Sadness is the emotion most of us will avoid feeling at all costs. Telling ourselves, 'It is for the best', when we endure a breakup, 'their loss' when we are passed over for that job or morphing sadness into anger as we swear at anyone crossing our path, might be the only way we can get through it. But when it is REALLY bad – death, cancer, divorce, disease bad – we don't always get the chance to reword sadness into something more palatable. We just have to sit in it. And that, as horrible as it feels, is what we need.

How to feel sad:

- **Say it out loud** – when we say it and hear it, the unknown element of fear about what is going on loosens its grip.

- **Feel what you feel** – that might even be nothing.

- **Know that two things can happen at once** – you can feel sad and still take your kids to school. That doesn't mean you aren't sad anymore or that you are 'over it'. It is just that the rhythm of life keeps going even when you really don't want it to.

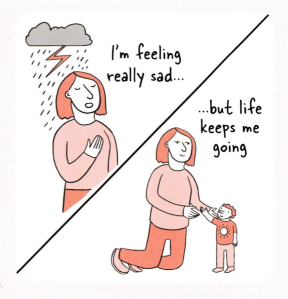

I'm feeling really sad...

...but life keeps me going

No emotion lasts forever.

Feeling sad means you care. And that means you will care again.

Bad

When the worst happens, we can be extremely hard on ourselves. We should have done more. Seen them more often. Asked more questions. Did what they asked of us even when we didn't want to. These feelings are another way of coping with difficult moments rather than feeling the pain. Our brains love a problem to solve and fix – if the outcome wasn't a good one, then why didn't we do more to fix it? This is an example of when your brain is talking nonsense. You did what you could with what you could at the time.

How to hold your own hand

Take a nap Being sad is mentally draining. A cat nap can recharge your battery just enough to help you begin to clean the lens (see page 122).

Watch something you love There is a reason they rerun eighties' comedies overnight and *White Christmas* every festive season. When we watch soothing shows or movies this can help us regulate our emotions, feel comforted and even just distract us from the difficult place that is our thoughts. You will have what works for you. (For me, it's *The Summer I Turned Pretty*.)

Take a walk Movement soothes our body and helps with oxygen and blood flow to our brain. It's never more needed than now.

Get outside From the sounds of nature to the smells of flowers (or food trucks) depending on where you live, these, along with a relaxed breathing pattern that often accompanies a short walk outside, can help tremendously.

Drink tea L-theanine, a botanical with stress reducing and calming properties fills every tea bag, along with brain supporting antioxidants which can support blood flow and brain health. And if you have someone to have a cup with, their company can be beneficial too.

Bake a cake Whether it is rice krispie cake or a five-layered iced sponge cake, the final outcome doesn't really matter. The process of recipe selection, ingredient hunting and then creating something with your own hands can help you see how capable you are of bringing joy. If it's delicious, even better.

Talk – or write – about it I had a patient once whose son killed himself. No warning, no note, no previous mental health issues. Nothing.

She told me she didn't want to talk about it. And then she would talk about it in every consultation we had for years afterwards, even if she was in to talk about something totally different. Everything always came back to her son.

When we talk about sad things to others who can listen to us, we connect. Their sadness becomes a memory or a feeling of our own sadness. We can find ways to put the pieces together differently about what has happened in our own minds.

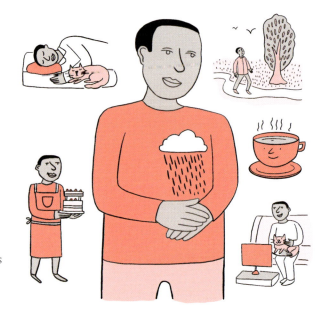

In the initial stages of the shit hitting the fan, venting and releasing what has happened in words is an essential strategy to survival. This is an essential download, but it's not the same as processing and coming to terms with what has happened and how you are feeling. It's important to know the difference and the benefits and limitations of each.

When or if you realise that continually venting isn't making you feel any lighter, it might be time to look at other ways to work through what has happened, including professional therapy.

If you can't or don't have someone to talk to, write it down.

Holding in sadness and negative feelings makes us sick.

Self-compassion

'I think part of the problem is that I hate myself.' Grace looked me straight in the eye and answered calmly when I asked her what she thought might be the reason she was so unhappy.

As tears filled both our eyes, I was struck by an ache of sadness from this woman who seemed so fine externally. A partner she loved, a toddler who slept through the night and a job as a nurse which was both fulfilling and the embodiment of all she'd worked for.

So what was the problem?

The good news was that Grace had taken the first step towards feeling better by making this admission. Realising on some level that part of why we feel as bad as we do during difficult times could be the way we see ourselves is a huge step forward. But how on earth do we do that?

When bad stuff happens, and unfortunately it will, we are more likely than ever to get into negative and harmful thought patterns as our brain tries to protect us from whatever has gone on in the outside world. When those negative thought patterns turn inward, they can really find a home and become ground into core until we can't really tell any more if it's just a fleeting thought or who we really are.

It's a weird thing that when something bad happens, too often we automatically take immediate responsibility or try to find the way we were implicit in making it happen.

Shame

We are our own harshest critics. When we need to stretch out the hand of friendship to ourselves, we don't. Hardwired to help us prevent such events occurring again as a method of survival, we turn inwards to shake ourselves into being different.

THAT WON'T WORK.

When we feel bad, asking ourselves why we did or didn't do something is only going to make us feel worse.

When I was diagnosed with MS, there were frequent nagging thoughts in my mind about why this had happened to me. Even as a doctor who knew the evidence about lack of clear causes, I was wracked with thoughts of *'If I'd gone to the doctor when I had that dizzy feeling, or that time I had numb feet, maybe things could have been different.'*

When we blame and shame ourselves for things that happen, we actively trigger an area of the brain, our amygdala, that prevents us from seeing all the facts. This area of our brain is key to emotional responses and making decisions. Therefore, when stressful thoughts occur in this way and their accompanying stress hormones are released, the amygdala is fighting against itself. By pointing the finger at ourselves, we are blocking our ability to see the bigger picture. Add into that some sleep deprivation, an external factor such as a toxic colleague, partner or an online post reaffirming these beliefs and we are on a slippery slope to self-loathing.

That isn't a good place to spend our time.

Remember our brains aren't designed to question how thoughts come. It tries to conserve energy for survival at all times, so when we think, *'I'm a complete disaster, no wonder I can't get a job / date / have a baby / look good in this outfit'*, we will believe it.

Grieving is tiring and studies have shown that it impacts our brain's ability to function – small things become huge and exhausting and our concentration and memory can be impacted.

When we quietly turn inwards during the tough times, there is another route we usually take to try to find our way out:

'THINGS HAPPEN FOR A REASON.'
'KEEP CALM AND CARRY ON.'

Are these positive, life-affirming statements to pull us up and through our tunnel of sadness? Or are they temporary sticking plasters that get us through the next hour / meeting / night until it all starts again?

The hard truth is that both are defence mechanisms designed to prop us up rather than rebuild at a foundational level.

For six years, I told almost no one about having MS. It felt shameful and like something I just needed to push through. So that's what I did. But health and mindset and mood don't work like that. Telling yourself you are bad doesn't work. And telling yourself 'You've got this' isn't that helpful either.

What does work?

Having compassion towards ourselves at all times, but especially in hard times, has been shown to help us learn from mistakes and the tough stuff and proactively make changes for the next time the walls fall in. When we treat ourselves in a nicer way, this helps with the release of oxytocin and feel-good brain chemicals. When we feel a bit better, surprise surprise, it is easier to have a more rounded view of what has happened and take proactive supportive steps to feel better. By doing this we actually deactivate our threat–defence system and instead, turn on a caring one.

Grace looked at me totally blankly when I tried to explain being kinder to herself. Then her daughter started crying during our appointment as she'd spilt glitter from her pen all over the surgery floor. Grace immediately hugged her and told her it didn't matter, it was only a bit of glitter and who didn't love some sparkle on their shoes? As they both started laughing and began scooping up the glitter massacre, I looked at Grace again, more tears filling my eyes and said 'Mummy saved the

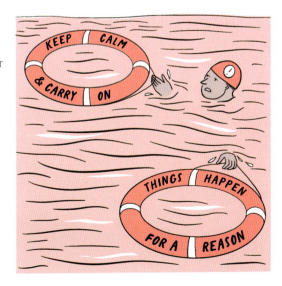

How to be kinder to yourself

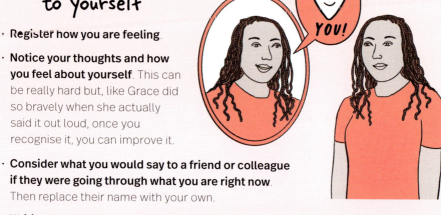

- **Register how you are feeling**.

- **Notice your thoughts and how you feel about yourself**. This can be really hard but, like Grace did so bravely when she actually said it out loud, once you recognise it, you can improve it.

- **Consider what you would say to a friend or colleague if they were going through what you are right now**. Then replace their name with your own.

- **Writing down how you feel helps**, and writing to yourself in the way you'd like a caring friend or relative to does too.

- **Don't wait for people to offer you sympathy and empathy**. It is always nice to get that support in these moments, but people don't really know how you are feeling. Only you do.

- **Say the things you want someone else to say but to yourself**. Like tying shoelaces and scrambling eggs, you have to learn the skill and keep practising.

day' thinking that the way she spoke to her daughter was exactly the way she could learn to speak to herself. I had no doubt she was like that with her patients too. It was the care for herself that she needed.

Grace smiled at me when she left in a way that told me, at least, in theory, she got it.

We are not designed to be nice to ourselves and hold our own hands. We are built to survive. But life isn't just about surviving so we have to teach ourselves ways to cope and feel better. And it all starts with caring for ourselves and knowing that when we are in our darkest deepest hole, this is what we need more than ever. Even if our thoughts are telling us something different.

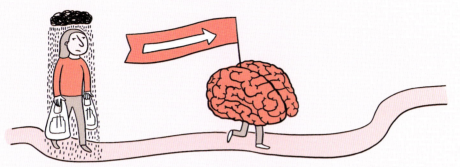

WHEN YOU FEEL THE WORST HAS HAPPENED...

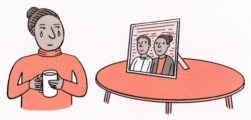

FACING YOUR SADNESS IS THE ONLY WAY TO MOVE THROUGH IT

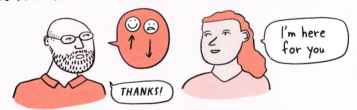

SHARING HOW YOU FEEL EASES THE LOAD

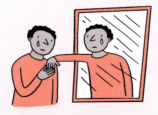

PLEASE BE KINDER TO YOURSELF

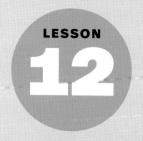
REST IN PEACE

IF ONLY I HAD . . .

'When do you think I will die, Doctor?'
More than one patient has asked me this – sometimes
in a setting of palliative care where there are signs the
end is almost in touching distance. But I've also been
asked this completely matter of factly on a Tuesday.
That one I didn't have an answer for.

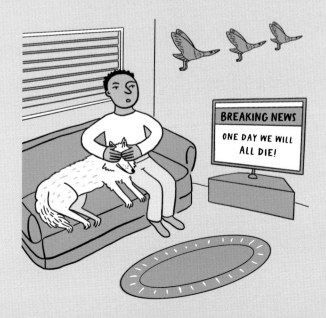

We see death on TV and movies and think of bloodshed, moments of great declaration and life-altering revelations.

Spoiler: in real life, most of the time death doesn't look or sound like that.

The outcome of a loved one dying will still be life-altering but by understanding more, we can hopefully reduce the shock and ideally prevent any bloodshed.

We have no control over how death meets us, but we can prepare ourselves and those we love for what matters to us in the end.

What happens when someone dies?

Natural dying is a process of shutting down, usually in the context of a serious illness and hopefully, old age.

Often there are signs that this process is taking place and when we understand this, it can be a way of helping ourselves prepare for what is probably going to happen. (I say 'probably' because while all the signs can point one way, we are all uniquely individual and there is no absolute protocol when it comes to anything in life, including death.)

This isn't to scare you or put you in a mindset of being a death detective, reviewing all your relatives' current state of health as if you were Columbo. It is to give an awareness and understanding of what the process of dying can look like. And once we have an idea of what may be happening, we can prepare ourselves a little bit better.

DYING ISN'T SCARY. THE THOUGHT OF LIVING WITHOUT SOMEONE IS.

Sad. Unfamiliar. Quiet. When someone nears the end of life, there is no time left to do any of the big things. But the most important moments are still to come.

What to expect when the end comes

The signals that this person is in the process of dying will often be there days or weeks before the end. While the final breath is the last one, the process of getting there is often slow and predictable when you know what to look for.

Physical changes – a reduction in appetite, slowing of mobility, sleeping more. The body is tired and doing what it needs to.

Mental / spiritual awareness – the person may talk more about people who have died, dream or have vivid memories of when their parents or other loved ones have died.

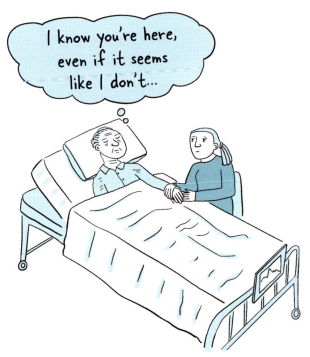

The final moments

Breath – the breathing pattern during dying has a particular name. As a junior doctor, when I was first called to the ward to someone who was 'Cheyne stoking', I was absolutely terrified. What was I supposed to do? The answer: *nothing*. Whether someone is going through this at home, in a hospice or on a ward, this is natural and with the right care, should be pain free.

(No) Speech – when we talk to someone, we are usually looking for answers or responses. When someone is dying, they are unlikely to respond with words that you might be expecting. They may say nothing at all. Talk, share, listen.

Heightened senses – while verbalising may not be possible, their sense of awareness is very likely still there. Studies have shown that hearing and touch are key senses that persist which is why many people choose to have music playing and keep a tender hand on a shoulder, arm or face.

Comfort – soothing a person during this process might sound like a job for a trained nurse and often, they can bring professionalism and reassurance to these moments that support everyone involved. But never underestimate what you can bring: as a relative or friend who cared for this person, your presence and kindness in these most important of moments can mean a lot.

What should I say? Whatever you feel you want to. If you want to make revelations or apologies, go ahead. But if you don't or can't, that's OK too. There is no space for regrets in a person's final moments. Your care and presence are all that matters, even if there were things you might think were left unsaid.

'I don't want to think about dying'
By avoiding talking about the hard stuff, we give it a shroud of uncertainty that breeds fear and allows us to imagine how horrible dying is. In reality, if we are lucky, we can help ourselves, and our loved ones, have the best death possible.

'What would you want in the end?'
A question we often never ask each other, or if we do it's when someone we love has just died and the emotions and whiskey are overflowing. But this is a question we can think of a plan for at any stage.

TALKING ABOUT DEATH DOESN'T MEAN IT'S GOING TO HAPPEN.

We hear a lot about manifesting – this is not like that. We take out insurance going on holiday or in our homes to plan for the possible eventuality of the worst thing happening, yet we know death will happen, but we avoid talking about it at all costs.

Let's change that.

Data has shown that when people with serious illnesses discuss their care with their clinicians and family, their suffering is less. Even if they move into hospice care sooner as was their wish, they actually survive longer.

The things we don't know:	What we do know:
When, how, whether we will have a life ending illness.	Death will happen.

Conversations to have with loved ones

If you imagined your last moments, where would you want them to be? Home, hospice, hospital?

Would you want anything particular with you – photos or music from times you've enjoyed?

Do you want to be cremated or buried?

How do you imagine your funeral? Where, what music do you want, should people wear black and drink tea or sparkle in glitter and pop the fizz to toast your life?

Power of Attorney forms

These exist for health circumstances to protect you in a stage where you might not be able to make your own decisions. They are empowering rather than depowering and hopefully, may never need to be used. But if you don't have one, and you become unable to make your own decisions, life for those around you becomes harder and there is no guarantee they will do what you would have wanted. If you haven't told them, how would they know?

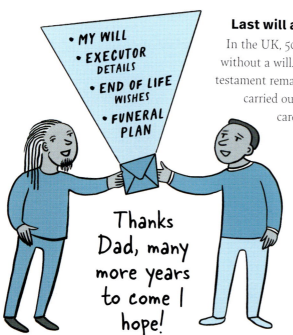

- MY WILL
- EXECUTOR DETAILS
- END OF LIFE WISHES
- FUNERAL PLAN

Thanks Dad, many more years to come I hope!

Last will and testament

In the UK, 50 per cent of people die without a will. This means your last will and testament remains unknown and cannot be carried out. You might think you don't care and what does it matter.

You matter. Your life's work and what you created and stood for matters.

Make a will today – these can be written for free.

You can amend it as circumstances and relationships alter throughout.

In the absence of this document, the law will decide what happens to your life's possessions. Think about that, all those decisions you angsted over in your lifetime, the shifts worked and jobs endured to make your life the best it could be. Whatever possessions you have deserve to be given or used in the way you want them to be. Regardless of whether those are diamonds or photo albums. It's not about the monetary value. It is about you and making sure your legacy serves what you've worked your whole life for.

Organ donation

In some countries, organ donation post-death is a standard process that occurs unless you have opted out in advance. If your family or loved ones are not aware of your decision, they can impact the outcome. This results in your wishes not being followed and stress and upset for family members.

This can be avoided by having these difficult conversations and being clear about what you do or definitely don't want.

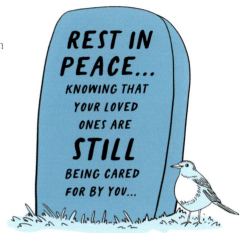

Expression of wishes

Not the same as a will, but what you want to happen with things that are important to you. Including your pension. No one wants their hard-earned pension going to the ex they divorced twenty years earlier but it you don't formally express your wishes, a default mechanism will kick in and that might end up with any assets, including those with sentimental value, ending up in the hands of people you didn't choose.

Why don't we talk about dying?

As a doctor, I saw my first dead body in my first week of work when I was twenty-two. Despite my training, I was emotionally unprepared for what I saw. Having recently attended a funeral for the first time where there was an open casket in my forties, I wondered how everyone would deal with this sight. As I watched young children approach the coffin, supported by older relatives, I became acutely aware that everyone in the room was in the sadness of grief and shock together. From the oldest to the youngest, there was a peculiar comfort in seeing everyone with the same sort of look across their face. The sight of a body in the coffin wasn't what people were weeping over, it was the loss of the life within it.

Apart from the obvious, I was interested to read that our own biases might be part of the reason we are death-talk avoidant. Consider these: Base rate bias: Even though death is the only certainty, because we feel fine, we think it won't happen to us. Normalcy bias: Because we haven't experienced it, we think it won't happen to us. Courtesy bias: We don't want to offend anyone, so we say the easy thing rather than the truth. Even doctors and nurses are guilty of this one: in a study of over 3,000 patients with metastatic breast cancer, only 16 per cent were given an accurate prognosis.

Talking about death and dying is hard. But when we don't talk about it, the outcomes are worse.

It's good to talk about death

Our brains crave routine and consistency. When we leave them to their own devices on any number of topics, they create stories and fill in the blanks themselves. Life ending is the only certainty we have. Many of the details around this remain unknown until then, but if we fill in as many blanks as we can, we can remove as much of the uncertainty as possible.

SHHH . . . WE WANT TO HEAR ABOUT DEATH.

Mitch Albom was a sports journalist who began interviewing a former professor of his to capture some of his essential wisdom as he neared the end of his life. He was so moved by the stories, he approached publishers about the prospect of a book. The book was rejected multiple times because 'talking about dying is a downer'. Nonetheless, *Tuesday's with Morrie* became the best-selling memoir of the twentieth century.

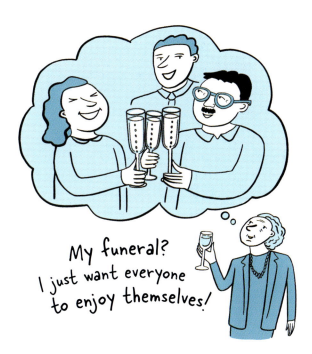

Death isn't just about you

We spend our lives caring and loving the people we choose. When death occurs there is a sadness and grief that can engulf us, sometimes for those that remain behind for the rest of their lives. If there is a way to make our own deaths easier on those we have spent our whole lives loving, it is to deal with the practical stuff that we can and leave some guidance about what we want when it happens. Let them remember us and love us in their own way, rather than obscuring those expressions of love and loss with legalities and technicalities.

Tragedies happen

There is no explanation or rationale for when death happens (although people will try desperately to give you one, whether you want it or not). The gut-wrenching, life-shattering impact of loss in this way is beyond comprehension. If you find yourself in this circumstance, and I hope you don't, remember that grief is not a condition to be treated or something you just need to get over.

It always sits with you: the loss becomes part of you, but it doesn't become you.

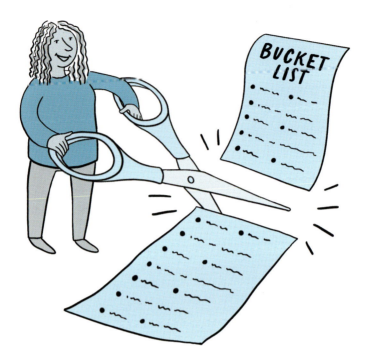

Make the list smaller

Whether you have a Bucket List, or Rainy-Day Fund , most people will have things they want to see, try or even accomplish in their lifetime. While the trip to the Grand Canyon may be something you talk about for the rest of your life, all the evidence points to the small things being the things that people feel most grateful for when they near the end of their life.

Strive for the goals that you set for yourself but know that this is for you and your current enjoyment. By giving weight to the everyday things that you take for granted when you are just all about living, when you can't do them anymore you will realise that those things are the one that give you the most enjoyment.

Grief

There is no timeline or straight line when it comes to grief. The impact of loss is more than sadness: it triggers the stress response which is an effort to protect us from further danger. The impact? Grief can cause disorientation and brain fog, as well as fatigue. This is you trying to make sense of what has happened, process this in some capacity and also protect yourself from further distress.

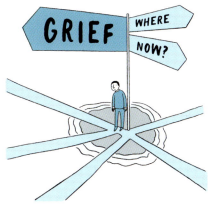

But it might help you to remember although this loss may feel insurmountable and that you will never see the sun again, we actually deal with loss every single day just on a much smaller scale. Life is full of endings. The carefree life of your twenties gave way to more responsibility in your thirties. Your freedom to do as you please ended if you became responsible for someone else. The boss that you looked up to and shaped your career retired. Mini loss is all around us and we always, always get through it in the end.

The big losses might take longer, and you will be different as a result but you, and your life, will carry on.

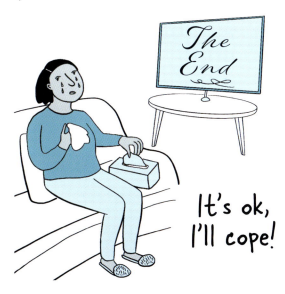

A sign of hope

Death remains the final ending that we are simultaneously working towards and avoiding at all costs. Signs of our loved ones can return in the most unexpected of places. My husband's brother died suddenly at the age of fifty-three. This was one of those life-shattering deaths that left an open wound so deep it was hard to imagine it could ever come back together. My sister-in-law turned to as many sources of comfort as she could in the months that followed, including feeding birds that came to visit in her garden. A single hungry robin returned day after day, even as the seasons changed. One day, having not left food out for some time, the robin reappeared and promptly took up position indoors under her coffee table. She told a neighbour about her new pet and was shocked when she was told that the robin was a sign of reassurance from the dead. Her son, a sceptical teenager, had his doubts, until the robin reappeared in the kitchen one day and took up a new comfortable residence, resting on his shoe.

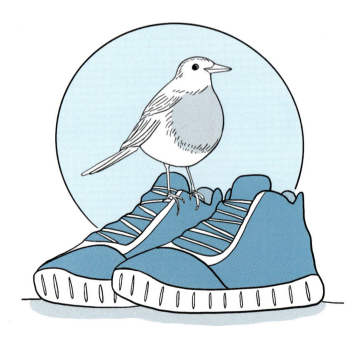

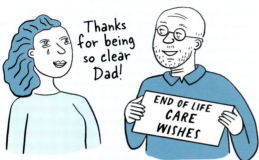

IT'S NEVER TOO EARLY TO TALK ABOUT WHAT YOU DO OR DON'T WANT WHEN YOU DIE

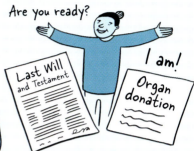

COMPLETE YOUR PAPERWORK AND ENCOURAGE OTHERS TO TOO

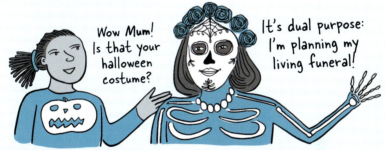

YOUR RELATIVES AND FRIENDS WILL HAVE ENOUGH TO DEAL WITH...

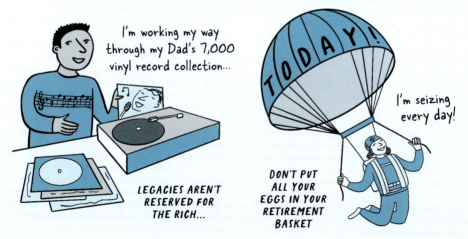

LEGACIES AREN'T RESERVED FOR THE RICH...

DON'T PUT ALL YOUR EGGS IN YOUR RETIREMENT BASKET

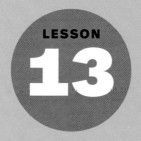

TIME, PURPOSE, INTENTION

'WHY DOES SATURDAY GO SO QUICKLY WHEN MATHS GOES SO SLOWLY?'
My son, aged 10

We live in fortunate times where we have scientists and researchers that are studying what makes us happy. Data collected over the last ninety years from the Harvard Study of Adult Development, one of the longest running studies of human happiness, has some pretty strong pointers about what matters in the end:

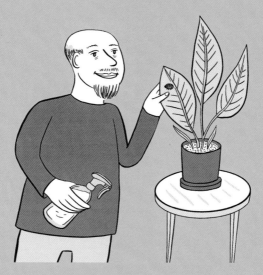

Meaningful social connections

That person or people you can ring at the end of a really horrid day and know that they will listen or perhaps offer you some advice that makes you feel better.

Who is that for you? Are you that person for someone else?

Working at and nurturing those relationships are at the core of a happy life that is well lived.

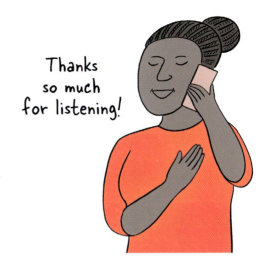

Staying engaged throughout our whole lives

This means recognising that what engages you and drives you at twenty won't be the same at sixty. And that's OK. The thing that matters is being engaged in something at all. While cognitive decline isn't inevitable as we age, how we think and see the world does alter. Our ability to innovate may reduce, working memory may not be as efficient so the old tasks may not be as easy as they were. That doesn't mean we can't learn and develop new skills on the back of a lifetime of experiences.

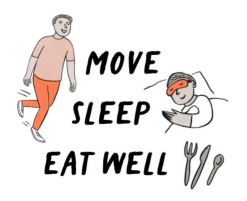

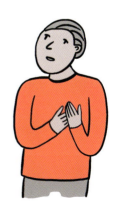

Paying attention to and respecting our bodies throughout our lifetime

We live in incredible vessels that break, rupture and hurt. But they are resilient and physical and even mental assaults can be healed. We have a part to play in this, too, however and caring for ourselves physically is important to stay the course for a long and happy life.

Move, sleep, eat with care and ask for help when pain, physical or mental, is not healing on its own.

Run your own race

Comparing achievements to our age and to those of our peers is how we are trained as children and young adults. But being top of the class doesn't matter any more at ten than it does as being the first to have a baby or pay a deposit for a flat at thirty.

'I wish I hadn't cared so much about what people thought of me' is one of the biggest regrets found by this *Harvard Study*, especially from women. Now that we can comment, like or dislike other people's lives on screens in real time, this will be an even harder challenge for our generation and the ones to come. But we owe it to ourselves and especially to the women who have spoken up before us to remember that we can fully control how we react to what people think of us.

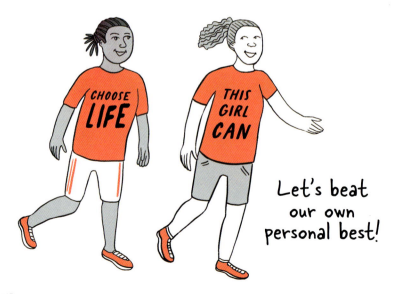

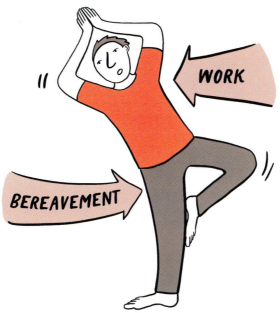

Balance

Often considered a boring concept but it is so important. Living our lives in the textbook way to ensure a happy and healthy existence isn't always possible. People die, hearts break, jobs harm you and what you have in your bank account will matter. You will lose your place in the story of your life more than once. It will take time to reset and get to where you need to be to continue.

This is why how we live and care for ourselves and our brain matters. By knowing how and why sleep matters, that sometimes we just need to do nothing when things are awful beyond belief or that being perimenopausal may be a strong reason you feel like nothing feels the same anymore, we can handle everything better.

Time

Maths goes slowly and weekends speed past us for a few different reasons. The dopamine hits our brain releases when we are having a good time can make it hard to quantify time as we are happily caught up in the moment. When time feels like it's achingly slow, it may be that our brain is trying to give the message that things aren't very fulfilling, and it is time to move on to something else. (I won't tell my son that one!)

The one constant I've heard patients say about the passage of time when they are facing a health issue or caring for a partner is that if they'd known that holiday / dinner out / visit to the grandkids was going to be their last 'as they were before', they'd have spent more time enjoying it.

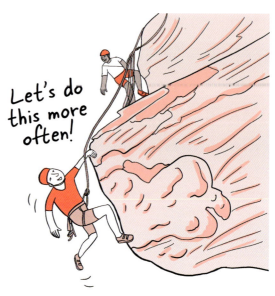

'I WISH WE COULD GO FOR JUST ONE MORE COFFEE WHEN SHE WAS THE WAY SHE USED TO BE.'

Most of us will not live outwardly extraordinary lives. Even with the best of intentions, we won't all create culture-changing tech, sell out stadiums or win a World Cup.

What matters is that we live our own version of an extraordinary life. And that is pretty much impossible to do if you are permanently tired, grumpy or fearful. Caring for your brain in the ways we have covered will facilitate you living in the way you deserve to. You get nothing for nothing as the well-known saying goes, and it's not easy to make changes to how you adapt and react to your surroundings. While your brain is geared up for change, it also doesn't really want you to make it. Conserving energy and maintaining your safety are its key purposes so to live and make change in the way you want or need to is hard. Resourcing yourself is essential to enable you to do this. What your brain consumes, both from the food you eat and the conversations you are part of, matters. Your brain is for survival not thinking so knowing its strengths and weaknesses is important.

I used to be a huge believer in superstition and fate. I thought that by experiencing so many difficult things through the eyes of my patients, this would somehow give me a repellent coating to avoid hard or bad things impacting me. As a GP, I had seen plenty of those moments, so I felt I had a big reserve to draw from when and if I needed it.

Now that I'm living with MS, I've changed my mind on all of that. (Thank you, neuroplasticity!)

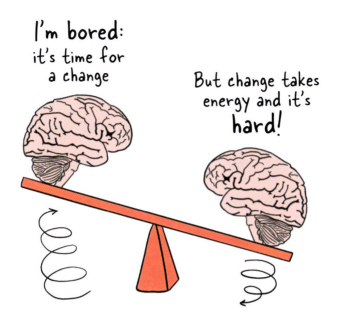

Life is a series of moments joined together by our own unique umbilical cord. As they are happening, we can enjoy the brilliant moments so much that we think they can erase and sustain us through the bad ones. But that isn't how it works. When we are grieving a loss, it's very hard to focus on purely the joy that that person brought to us. Similarly, when we are crying with joy at a moment of peak accomplishment or small victory, replacing that brightness with a shutter of dark would be unthinkable.

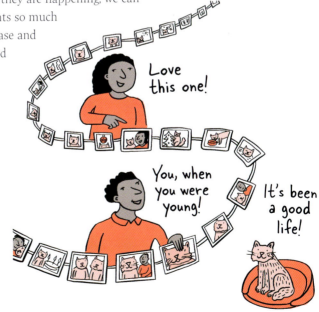

Think about how much time and focus you put into planning a holiday or a weekend away. Those experiences can be brilliant, but I don't think I'm alone in thinking that sometimes, holidays aren't all they are cracked up to be. Travel is delayed, someone gets sick, the weather is not what you were expecting. And then what? We've invested so much of ourselves in making these few days the perfect break that we needed and as is often the case, it just didn't work out as you planned. Imagine if we decided to put even more of that energy into caring for our brains on an everyday basis as opposed to pinning our hopes on a week in the sunshine being the fix-all?

The secret lies in holding each moment, good, bad or just a delicious coffee on a Thursday, for exactly what it is. And not being so exhausted, sad or anxious that you overblow it or, even worse, miss it all together.

Your brain will help you get your body to Friday in one piece, but you can influence how that day goes, and the one after that.

By caring for our brains in small ways every day, we are ensuring we have our foundational corner pieces in place. So, when life throws us the next part of our puzzle to complete, it's easier to see the whole picture.

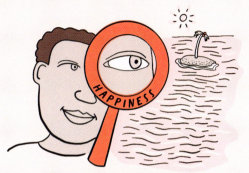

DESPERATELY SEEKING HAPPINESS ALMOST GUARANTEES YOU WILL RARELY FIND IT

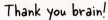
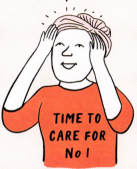

FOCUS ON YOUR OWN BRAINCARE

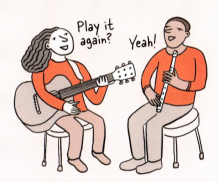

WHO WE SPEND OUR TIME WITH...

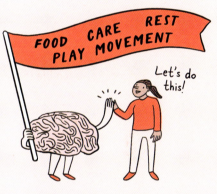

WITH FUEL CARE REST...

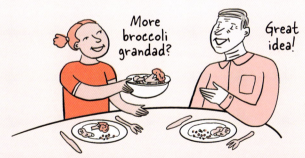

YOU ARE NEVER TOO YOUNG OR OLD TO BEGIN CARING FOR YOUR BRAIN

FURTHER READING

STOP LOOK LISTEN
'Do Pause' Robert Poynton

SLEEP NAP REST
https://www.sleepfoundation.org/insomnia/treatment/cognitive-behavioral-therapy-insomnia

WRITE SING DRAW
'Big Magic' Elizabeth Gilbert

COOK FEED NOURISH
'This is Your Brain on Food' Dr Uma Naidoo

QUIT RUN HIDE
'Fierce Self Compassion' Dr Kristin Neff

YOU ME THEM
'Maybe you should talk to someone' Lori Gottlieb

WALK RUN BOOGIE
Give this playlist a listen: *Heads Up* - WalkRunBoogie
https://open.spotify.com/playlist/3Op7fymsrCjbx15lBNa1Lk?si=gRr31VKfQGGWpHhntwTi8g

TICK TOCK BOOM
'The XX Brain' Lisa Mosconi

LAUGH GIGGLE PLAY
'Laughology' Stephanie Davies

FEEL CRY FROWN
'Permission to Feel' Professor Marc Brackett

SAD BAD SURVIVAL
'Love for Imperfect Things' Haemin Sunam

REST IN PEACE
'With the End in Mind' Dr Kathryn Mannix

TIME PURPOSE INTENTION
'Peace is Every Breath' Thich Nhat Hanh

ACKNOWLEDGEMENTS

Thank you to my patients, who have taught me everything I've learned about health and wellbeing. Being a doctor is a true privilege and from this, I've seen the importance of truly listening to each other which, in turn, has helped me put the pieces together when it comes to brain care.

Writing is the thing that 10 year old me always wanted to do, so being able to combine this with my Doctor life is a dream come true. Thank you to my agent Silé Edwards who answers all my questions with kindness and is a constant source of support. Thanks also to Sophie, Charlotte and the team at Quarto books.

Finally, thank you to my husband for encouraging me to keep going, and to my son, who inspires me and makes me laugh every day.

Quarto

First published in 2025 by Leaping Hare Press
an imprint of The Quarto Group.
One Triptych Place, London, SE1 9SH
United Kingdom
T (0)20 7700 9000
www.Quarto.com

EEA Representation, WTS Tax d.o.o., Žanova ulica 3, 4000 Kranj, Slovenia

Text © 2025 Dr Clara Doran
Illustrations © 2025 Sandra Howgate
Design © 2025 Quarto Publishing Plc

ISBN 978-1-83600-477-6
EBOOK ISBN 978-1-83600-478-3

10 9 8 7 6 5 4 3 2 1

Book Designer: Sally Bond
Commissioning Editor: Sophie Lazar
Editorial Director: Jenny Barr
Publisher: Monica Perdoni
Senior Designer: Renata Latipova
Senior Editor: Charlotte Frost
Senior Production Controller: Rohana Yusof

Printed in China

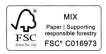